# Acknowledgments

KW-178-083

This project demonstrated, like most worthwhile things in life, that we are dependent on each other and our sum is much greater than our parts. Without the following people, this book would not have existed. Thank you!

Linda Savage and Diane Lamsback—your untiring efforts and skills drove this project.

Toby, Mags, Lizzie, Ellie, and my wife, Kate, the loves of my life—thank you for putting up with dining room tables filled with manuscripts and a sometimes preoccupied father/husband.

Bill "The Dude" Dexter—you almost left us. Glad you are still around man. You continue to show us how to *really* live! Muchas gracias, compadré. Jay Smith, Lev Nazarian, and Jon Jacobson—you started the revolution and cleared the path! The chapter authors, all outstanding clinicians and MSK ultrasound gurus—you showed us the way! Our students, residents, and fellows—you are our future!

Ancora Imparo!

James M. Daniels

Many thanks to my fellows, past, present, and future, who give me direction and purpose and joy in what I do. Special thanks to Hatz and Kate. There is a lot of both of you in this book. And to my lovely and patient wife, Cindy, and our children, Ben, Sam, and Hannah, on whom I practiced my ultrasound skills and with whom I will now surely move on to the next adventure.

William W. Dexter

# Basics of Musculoskeletal Ultrasound

## DATE DUE

| | | | |
|---|---|---|---|
| | | | |
| | | | |
| | | | |
| | | | |
| | | | |
| | | | |
| | | | |
| | | | |
| | | | |
| | | | |
| | | | |
| | | | |
| | | | |
| | | | |
| | | | |
| | | | |
| | | | |
| | | | PRINTED IN U.S.A. |

Basics of Musculoskeletal Ultrasound

James M. Daniels • William W. Dexter

Editors

# Basics of Musculoskeletal Ultrasound

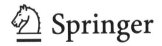 Springer

*Editors*

James M. Daniels, MD, MPH, FAAFP,
    FACOEM, FACPM
Departments of Family and Community Medicine
Department of Orthopedic Surgery
Southern Illinois University School of Medicine
Quincy, IL, USA

William W. Dexter, MD, FACSM
Sports Medicine and Family Medicine
Maine Medical Center
Tufts University School of Medicine
Portland, ME, USA

ISBN 978-1-4614-3214-2        ISBN 978-1-4614-3215-9 (eBook)
DOI 10.1007/978-1-4614-3215-9
Springer New York Heidelberg Dordrecht London

Library of Congress Control Number: 2013934108

Printed on acid-free paper

Springer is part of Springer Science+Business Media (www.springer.com)

# Contents

# Contributors

**Erik Adams** Midwest Sports Institute, Middleton, WI, USA

**Joseph J. Albano** Department of Regenerative Medicine, Comprehensive Orthopedics and Sports Medicine, Salt Lake City, UT, USA

**Matthew C. Bayes** Crane Clinic for Sports Medicine, Chesterfield, MO, USA

**James M. Daniels** Departments of Family and Community Medicine and Orthopedic Surgery, Southern Illinois University School of Medicine, Quincy, IL, USA

**Kevin deWeber** Department of Family Medicine, Uniformed Services University of the Health Sciences, Bethesda, MD, USA

**William W. Dexter** Sports Medicine and Family Medicine, Maine Medical Center, Tufts University School of Medicine, Portland, ME, USA

**Pierre d'Hemecourt** Division of Sports Medicine, Primary Care Sports Medicine, Boston Children's Hospital, Boston, MA, USA

**Joshua G. Hackel** University of West Florida, Pensacola, FL, USA

Primary Care Sports Medicine, The Andrews Institute, Gulf Breeze, FL, USA

**John Hatzenbuehler** Department of Family Medicine, Maine Medical Center, Portland, ME, USA

**John Charles Hill** Family Medicine and Sports Medicine, University of Colorado School of Medicine, Denver, CO, USA

**Allyson S. Howe** Department of Family Medicine, Maine Medical Center, Portland, ME, USA

**Anthony E. Joseph** Portneuf Medical Center, Pocatello Orthopaedic and Sports Medicine Institute/Idaho State University, Pocatello, ID, USA

**Mark E. Lavallee** South Bend-Notre Dame Sports Medicine Fellowship Program, South Bend, IN, USA

Department of Family Medicine, Indiana University School of Medicine, Indianapolis, IN, USA

Memorial Hospital of South Bend and Memorial Medical Group, South Bend, IN, USA

Indiana University South Bend, South Bend, IN, USA

Holy Cross College, South Bend, IN, USA

University of Notre Dame, Men's Soccer Team, South Bend, IN, USA

USA Weightlifting, Sports Medicine Society, Colorado Springs, CO, USA

Division of Sports Medicine, Department of Family Medicine, Memorial Hospital of South Bend, South Bend, IN, USA

**Matthew S. Leiszler** Family Medicine and Sports Medicine, University of Colorado School of Medicine, Denver, CO, USA

**Linda Savage** Department of Family and Community Medicine, SIU School of Medicine, Quincy, IL, USA

**Patrick A. Smith** Department of Orthopaedic Surgery, University of Missouri Hospitals and Clinics, Columbia, MO, USA

Columbia Orthopaedic Group, Columbia, MO, USA

**J. Herbert Stevenson** Departments of Family and Community Medicine and Orthopedics and Rehabilitation, University of Massachusetts Medical Center, University of Massachusetts Medical School, Worcester, MA, USA

**Ralf G. Thiele** Division of Allergy/Immunology and Rheumatology, Department of Medicine, University of Rochester, Rochester, NY, USA

**Matt E. Thornburg** Columbia Orthopaedic Group, Columbia, MO, USA

University of Missouri, Columbia, MO, USA

**Paul D. Tortland** Valley Sports Physicians and Orthopaedic Medicine, Avon, CT, USA

# Introduction

James M. Daniels and William W. Dexter

Clinical ultrasonography has been around for decades. In Europe, it also has been used for many years, but the way it is utilized differs from the system developed in North America.

In Europe, ultrasound scanning is introduced to medical students very early in their training. These skills are then supplemented in postgraduate training. In the United States, clinical examination skills are taught to all students, but very few are exposed to clinical ultrasonography. Traditionally, a clinician examines the patient, and if it is determined that an ultrasound study is necessary, a comprehensive scan is performed by a highly trained technician, a sonographer. The images are then interpreted by a highly trained physician, a radiologist, who then generates a detailed report back to the clinician. This paradigm has shifted slightly over the years, with cardiologists and obstetricians using ultrasound as a bedside tool to practice medicine, but this training is limited in scope and is only taught in residency or fellowship. Recently, the United States has adopted a hybrid of these two systems, referred to as "point-of-care" ultrasonography. Students and practicing clinicians are now being trained to use bedside ultrasound as an important tool to diagnose and treat patients (i.e., starting central lines in the ICU, FAST scans in the Emergency Department, dynamic scanning of shoulder joint).

This model integrates the history and physical exam along with treatment decisions into one process by one clinician. It not only decreases the cost and time of the process, it allows the clinician to evaluate three-dimensional real-time anatomy and physiology, which further adds to the accuracy of the diagnosis. These "point-of-care" musculoskeletal ultrasound studies (POC MSK/US) may or may not always include the "comprehensive" evaluation that traditional ultrasound examinations do, depending on the reason they were performed. These scans are to supplement the clinical examination and should not be used as a stand-alone way to diagnose the patient's condition. The use of the ultrasound machine can be compared to the use of a stethoscope in the clinical setting. The stethoscope, as we know it, was first used in France in the early 1800s by Dr. René Laennec, but it wasn't widely used until the mid-1900s, when Rappaport and Sprague were able to mass-produce a lightweight, relatively affordable model. Ultrasound technology is currently following this trend. We predict that POC US will be the stethoscope of the twenty-first century. In fact, the year 2013 has been heralded as "The Year of Sonography" by a number of health-care organizations. The use of POC US has vastly changed the way musculoskeletal medicine is being practiced today and will transform the way we practice in the future.

We propose to use an ultrasound machine as one would a stethoscope—to no longer view it as a test to be ordered but as an extension of the physical examination. Most textbooks on this subject are written by radiologists with years of experience in the traditional paradigm described above. This book is written by busy clinicians with decades of experience using clinical ultrasound and could be used as a stand-alone curriculum for POC MSK/US.

This book is laid out in a way to become a bedside aid to assist in POC MSK/US scanning. Each chapter emphasizes one particular skill set. Introduction chapters demonstrate knobology, tissue scanning techniques, and the certification/accreditation process for MSK/US. Later chapters concentrate on particular regions of the body. The main focus of each chapter revolves around a table that shows probe positions, patient positioning, surface anatomy, and underlying structures to be scanned. A small amount of text accompanies each table, but this book focuses on clinical exam skills. A list

J.M. Daniels, M.D., MPH (✉)
Departments of Family and Community Medicine and Orthopedic Surgery,
Southern Illinois University School of Medicine,
612 North 11th Street, Quincy, IL 62301, USA
e-mail: jdaniels@siumed.edu

W.W. Dexter, M.D., FACM
Sports Medicine and Family Medicine, Maine Medical Center,
Tufts University School of Medicine,
272 Congress Street, Portland, ME 04101, USA
e-mail: dextew@mmc.org

J.M. Daniels and W.W. Dexter (eds.), *Basics of Musculoskeletal Ultrasound*,
DOI 10.1007/978-1-4614-3215-9_1, © Springer Science+Business Media New York 2013

of "red flags," potentially serious conditions to consider, and "clinical pearls" or tips to improve scanning techniques is also included. We have also included a number of clinical exercises or "homework" that can be used to improve and document your scanning skills. A "check-off" list of important structures to evaluate is also provided along with some examples of sample reports.

Many other references are available to explain detailed anatomy and scanning techniques. Please refer to them if needed. This book was developed to be used at bedside and to assist in scanning. Many of the chapter authors of this book also teach POS MSK/US. When we asked them what was the best advice they could give clinicians who want to incorporate these skills in their practice, they gave three recommendations: "PRACTICE! PRACTICE! PRACTICE!"

Although this book can be used at a POC MSK/US training course, it is designed to assist clinicians to scan. If one waits until one has "perfect" technique and all the anatomy memorized, one will never be able to fully utilize this technology. These skills are integrative, not additive. The use of MSK/US will not only decrease the cost but also increase the effectiveness of treatment (the definition of high quality of health care proposed by some experts). In addition, it allows us to touch our patients, which has been shown to increase both patient and provider satisfaction when it comes to providing health care.

# Understanding Accreditation and Certification in Musculoskeletal Ultrasound

Joshua G. Hackel

## What Is the Difference Between Accreditation and Certification for Musculoskeletal Ultrasound?

It is important to understand the essential differences between accreditation and certification.

### Accreditation

The term "accreditation" is typically used to refer to practices, not people. Therefore, a person or group of people can choose to have their practice "accredited" by a recognized accrediting body. The accrediting body awards practice accreditation to those practices that adhere to certain standards. The standards themselves may vary among different organizations but would generally include language concerning the qualifications of the people performing in that practice, the equipment used (type and maintenance), and the logistics of the practice (patient scheduling, documentation, use of protocols, emergency plans, etc.). Common examples would be fellowship accreditation by the American College of Graduate Medical Education (ACGME) or hospital accreditation by the Joint Commission on the Accreditation of Health Care Organizations (JCAHO).

### Certification

The term "certification" is typically used to refer to people/individuals and not practices. Therefore, a person may

become certified in a field or technique by demonstrating that he or she has met specific standards. For the most part, this includes documentation of prerequisites (e.g., Continuing Medical Education [CME] and/or years of experience) and passing some type of test (written and/or practical). Individual certification may be used to document an individual's competency in support of an application for practice accreditation, but practice accreditation will not typically suffice to obtain certification. The obvious example is that many, if not most, American Medical Society for Sports Medicine (AMSSM) members are "certified" in sports medicine once they meet the prerequisites (e.g., completion of fellowship) and pass the test that is managed by an outside institution (Board of Medical Examiners).

## What Organizations Have Set Up a System for Accreditation and Certification?

### Accreditation

Practice accreditation for musculoskeletal ultrasound (MSK/US) is currently available through the American Institute of Ultrasound in Medicine (AIUM). The AIUM is a nonprofit, multidisciplinary organization dedicated to advancing safe and effective use of ultrasound in medicine through professional and public education, research, development of guidelines, and practice accreditation. Although the AIUM promotes all types of US, the organization has recently focused on the emerging field of MSK/US, supporting guideline development, education, advocacy, and, of course, practice accreditation. The AIUM has a long history of practice accreditation and is recognized as a legitimate accrediting organization by CMS and third-party payers. At this time, AIUM practice accreditation is the only available practice accreditation in MSK/US. You do not have to be a member of the AIUM to have the AIUM accredit your practice. We are currently not aware of any other organizations developing practice accreditation in MSK/US. If you are

J.G. Hackel, M.D. (✉)
University of West Florida, Gulf Breeze, FL, USA

Primary Care Sports Medicine, The Andrews Institute,
1040 Gulf Breeze Parkway, Suite 200, Gulf Breeze, FL 32561, USA
e-mail: joshua.hackel@bhcpns.org

J.M. Daniels and W.W. Dexter (eds.), *Basics of Musculoskeletal Ultrasound*,
DOI 10.1007/978-1-4614-3215-9_2, © Springer Science+Business Media New York 2013

interested in learning more about the AIUM and practice accreditation, go to http://www.aium.org, the official web site of the AIUM.

## Certification

Individual certification for MSK/US is under development by two organizations. There is certification being developed by the American Registry for Diagnostic Medical Sonography (ARDMS). The ARDMS is a nonprofit organization that promotes quality care and patient safety through the certification and continuing competency of ultrasound professionals. Similar to the AIUM, the ARDMS is a well-established organization recognized by CMS and third-party payers as a legitimate certifying/credentialing certification. In fact, most sonographers you know have received one or more credentials (or certificates) from the ARDMS—for example, Registered Diagnostic Medical Sonographer (RDMS) and Registered Vascular Technologist (RVT). The ARDMS has developed a written test for MSK/US that is available to sonographers and physicians. This is a 200-question multiple-choice test that was developed by a multidisciplinary group of MSK/US experts. The final prerequisites for the ARDMS test are the following:

The applicant must

1. Hold an active certification or license in a health-related field
2. Required clinical MSK/US experience
   (a) Possess a minimum of 150 MSK/US studies that are performed and/or interpreted/reported within the preceding 36 months of application
3. Continuing Medical Education
   (a) ARDMS recommends and encourages applicants to earn a minimum of 30 MSK ultrasound specific CME's to assist in prepartion for the exam. This however is not a requirement
4. Documentation required with application
   (a) Copy of current valid license or active certification in a health-related field
   (b) Completed online self-attestation form indicating that you have performed and/or interpreted/reported a minimum of 150 MSK/US studies within the preceding 36 months before applying
   (c) A patient log indicating that you have performed/interpreted/reported a minimum of 150 MSK/US studies. This log does not need to be submitted with the application but may be requested as part of a random audit. This documentation should be maintained by the applicant for at least 36 months following the date of application for the MSK examination
5. Provide a photocopy of a non-expired government-issued photo identification with signature; the name on the identification must exactly match the name under which you are applying for ARDMS examination. Include documentation of CME in MSK/US and practice experience. AMSSM members interested in learning more about the ARDMS and MSK/US certification should go to http://www.ardms.org, the official web site of the ARDMS

It should be noted that the AIUM and ARDMS are, in a sense, "sister" organizations that complement, not compete, with each other. This is similar to the ACGME and the Board of Medical Examiners. The American College of Rheumatology is also developing a certification process for rheumatologists who perform MSK/US.

## What Is the Timeline for Accreditation and Certification to Start?

AIUM practice accreditation for MSK/US was initiated July 2010 and therefore is currently available. ARDMS certification in MSK/US was initiated September 2012.

## What Are the Standards and Guidelines for the Accreditation of Ultrasound Practices?

The AIUM web site has very detailed information on this process: http://www.aium.org/accreditation/gettingStarted. AIUM practice accreditation is based largely upon the published AIUM guidelines for Performance of the Musculoskeletal Examination and Qualifications for Performing the MSK/US Examination, both available for free at the AIUM web site. The accreditation application includes sections in which the practice documents compliance with these guidelines. In addition, practices are required to list the different locations in which scanning is performed, who performs the scanning, which US machines are used, what type of US machine maintenance schedule is in place, what scanning protocols are utilized, how patients are scheduled, and how studies are documented in a timely manner. Practice guidelines for the performance of MSK/US as well as training guidelines are also included on this site for free.

## What Are the AIUM Practice Guidelines for the Performance of the Musculoskeletal Examination?

These are available on the AIUM web site and are free. They can be viewed at this link: http://www.aium.org/publications/guidelines/musculoskeletal.pdf.

## What Are the Current AIUM Training Guidelines for Physicians Who Evaluate and Interpret Musculoskeletal Ultrasound Exams?

These are available on the AIUM web site and are free. They can be viewed at this direct link: http://www.aium.org/publications/viewStatement.aspx?id=41.

Key items that are pertinent are noted below. You should familiarize yourself with the full document on the web site. In summary, a number of pathways can be taken:

- Completion of a residency or fellowship program supervised by a physician qualified to perform MSK/US examinations that provides structured MSK/US training, including the performance, interpretation, and reporting of 150 MSK/US examinations. The applicant will also need to have completed 40 h of AMA PRA Category 1 Credits specific to MSK/US, including at least one MSK/US course that includes hands-on training unless within 2 years of completion of a residency and/or fellowship.
  Or
- Completion of an ACGME- or AOA-accredited residency in a specialty practice plus 100 h of AMA PRA Category 1 Credits in MSK medicine, surgery, and/or imaging, of which at least 40 h need to be specific to MSK/US, including at least one MSK/US course that includes hands-on training, supervision and/or performance, interpretation, and reporting of 150 MSK/US examinations within the last 36 months. Completion of 60 h of non-MSK/US-specific CME if they are within 2 years of residency and/or fellowship training in a specialty that focuses on MSK medicine and/or surgery.

## Maintenance of Competence

All physicians performing MSK/US examinations should demonstrate evidence of continuing competence in the interpretation and reporting of those examinations. A minimum of 50 diagnostic MSK/US examinations per year is recommended to maintain the physician's skills.

## Continuing Medical Education

The physician should complete 30 h of AMA PRA Category 1 Credits specific to MSK/US every 3 years.

## What Are the Case Study Submission Requirements for AIUM Certification?

Practices will need to submit five cases for review by experts identified by the AIUM staff. These five cases should be representative of your practice. If the practice is a solo practice, then all cases can come from one clinician. However, if more than one person is scanning in the practice, then cases should come from multiple individuals. Similarly, if the practice evaluates all body regions, then the practice should not submit five shoulder examinations. For each case, the practice will submit all the US pictures and the report. The submitted pictures should comply with AIUM scanning protocols (i.e., Guidelines for Performance of the MSK/US Examination) and be labeled appropriately. The reports should justify the indication for the examination, and the stated results should accurately reflect the submitted US pictures. The AIUM has a well-established protocol for managing the process within HIPAA guidelines.

## How Much Will Accreditation and Certification Approximately Cost?

AIUM practice accreditation is approximately $1,000. The cost for the ARDMS MSK/US test is available on the ARDMS web site.

## Do I Need to Get Certified for Payment from Insurance Companies?

Neither practice accreditation nor personal certifications are necessarily tied to reimbursement. As outlined in their mission statements, the primary goals of the ARDMS and AIUM are to ensure best practices and patient safety. An analogy would be board certification in sports medicine. You certainly don't need to be certified in sports medicine to get reimbursed. The primary purpose of the sports medicine board is to ensure best practices in sports medicine; the board was not developed to ensure reimbursement. There is some precedent for CMS and third-party payers to utilize certification and practice accreditation to control patient access and reimbursement. For example, some insurance companies will not pay for imaging done at nonaccredited imaging centers, whereas others may only reimburse interventional spinal procedures performed by specialist's board certified in pain medicine. The reality is that practice accreditation and certification does set a minimum standard that third-party payers may utilize to ensure a minimum standard of care for their patients. Above and beyond the issue of reimbursement, there may be implications for marketing. Practices have certainly utilized specialty certifications and practice accreditations to distinguish themselves from competitors as part of a marketing strategy. Only time will tell how accreditation and certification will impact patient access and reimbursement.

## Do Accreditation and Certification Bodies Handle Diagnostic Ultrasound and Ultrasound for Needle Guidance Procedures Differently?

At this current time, the practice accreditation process pertains to diagnostic ultrasound. This means that practices should submit diagnostic ultrasound cases for review as part of their accreditation application. Although not specifically stated, it may be assumed that a practice accredited in MSK/US is accredited for diagnostic and interventional aspects. The AIUM has plans to develop practice guidelines for US-guided interventional procedures. How this will impact the MSK/US accreditation process remains to be determined. Based on our current understanding, the ARDMS certification test is primarily, if not entirely, diagnostic. The emphasis on diagnostic ultrasound for practice accreditation and certification is in line with the general understanding that individuals using US for US-guided procedures should have a basic understanding of diagnostic US. This reflects the European experience in which many clinicians are not taught US-guided procedures until they have met minimum requirements for diagnostic US.

## Suggested Reading

Bianchi S, Martinoli C. Ultrasound of the musculoskeletal system. New York, NY: Springer; 2007.

European Society of Musculoskeletal Radiology at their web site: http://www.essr.org/cms/website.php?id=/en/essr_home.htm.

# Choosing Ultrasound Equipment

**3**

Paul D. Tortland

## Introduction

Choosing an ultrasound system for musculoskeletal work can be a daunting task. With an increasing number of ultrasound vendors, each potentially offering a wide array of models with varying features, making a choice can be a challenge. A frequently asked question by those new to musculoskeletal ultrasound is, "What system should I buy?" That's akin to someone asking, "What car should I buy?" The simple answer is, "It depends."

## Console vs. Portable

The first choice is whether to purchase a cart-based console system or a portable system.

Console systems are generally large-format cart units. Their main advantage lies in their processing power. The bigger platform allows for more powerful processors and cooling fans. This translates into potentially better images and the ability to drive a wider array of transducers. Most also have the capacity to keep multiple transducers plugged in simultaneously, simplifying the process of switching between them.

While mobile (the carts all have casters), the size of console systems limits the ability to move them easily from room to room. Most do not have battery backup, which means that the unit must be fully powered down, unplugged, moved to the new location, and then plugged back in and rebooted. Most offices utilizing console systems, therefore,

will dedicate a room to ultrasound, where the system takes up more or less permanent residence.

For those new to musculoskeletal ultrasound, console systems have one major drawback. They cannot be taken home easily, which means that the user is limited to using the machine only while in the office. This can significantly hamper learning, because, let's face it, most of us do not want to stay late after a long day of seeing patients to practice on the ultrasound machine.

Portable machines, on the other hand, have the distinct advantage of, well, portability! The majority have battery backup built in, allowing the unit to be moved freely among exam rooms without having to power down each time. The portability also means the physician can take the unit home to practice, thereby significantly improving one's skills much more quickly.

Portable machines lack the processing power of the console systems, but for all but the most demanding applications, this is not a serious drawback. Portable units can easily handle the vast majority of musculoskeletal work.

Most portable systems lack the ability to plug in multiple transducers simultaneously. To change transducers, the operator must unplug one transducer and plug in another. On those systems in which the transducer plugs into the bottom of the machine, changing transducers can be more cumbersome or difficult.

If a portable machine is purchased, serious consideration should be given also to purchasing a mobile stand or a *docking cart*. A mobile stand holds the machine securely during use. Most also have various shelves for peripherals such as thermal image printers, CD burners, and holders for transducers. A docking cart, on the other hand, is a powered mobile stand into which the machine slides or docks, similar to a laptop docking station. It allows peripherals and several transducers to remain plugged into the cart; all you do is snap in/out the ultrasound machine.

Stands and carts make it easier to move the machine around the office but also make it much less likely that the

P.D. Tortland, D.O. (✉)
Valley Sports Physicians and Orthopaedic Medicine,
54 West Avon Road, Suite 202, Avon, CT 06001, USA
e-mail: Ptortland@gmail.com

J.M. Daniels and W.W. Dexter (eds.), *Basics of Musculoskeletal Ultrasound*,
DOI 10.1007/978-1-4614-3215-9_3, © Springer Science+Business Media New York 2013

machine will fall off an exam table or counter. The cost of a stand is a small insurance premium. In addition, some stands, and most docking carts, have the ability to keep more than one transducer plugged in at the same time, and the choice of which transducer is active is made via the keyboard. (Keep in mind, however, that depending on the system you choose, not all attached transducers may be accessible while the system is operating in battery mode.)

## Transducer Choices

For musculoskeletal work, the workhorse transducer is the linear probe. The ideal multipurpose transducer should have a frequency range of roughly 8–12 MHz. The vast majority of musculoskeletal ultrasound work is done at 10 MHz, with a smattering at 12 MHz for the more superficial structures (within 2-cm depth) and some at 8 MHz for slightly deeper structures (4–5-cm depth).

Some newer systems offer linear transducers that will scan at frequencies from 8 MHz to as high as 15–18 MHz. However, note that, depending on the particular system, you may not be able to choose the specific scanning frequency. Also, keep in mind that while a higher-frequency transducer may generate a higher-resolution image, it does so at the potentially heavy cost of severely limiting penetration or scanning depth, often to no more than 2 cm. (Remember that frequency and penetration are inversely related.)

Although the majority of work done in musculoskeletal ultrasound is handled by the linear transducer, strong consideration should be given also to purchasing a curved transducer with a frequency range of roughly 3–5 MHz. The curved arrays are essential for work around the hip and buttocks (including hip intra-articular injections and piriformis trigger point injections) and spine work. However, curved probes can also be extremely helpful in other areas, such as the anterior glenohumeral joint (which is relatively deep and not well visualized by most linear arrays), or in cases of large or obese patients, where the linear transducer lacks the penetration. Finally, curved transducers can be helpful to start out getting a wider field of view of an area, for example, to help localize a tear in a muscle belly, and then the linear probe can be used to "zoom in" on the affected area.

A wide assortment of specialized probes is also available, such as small-footprint "hockey stick" probes, small low-frequency curved arrays, and dedicated high-frequency probes. These specialized probes may be useful in practices or specialties that tend to do highly specialized ultrasound. For example, for rheumatologists who use ultrasound extensively to examine and inject the small joints of the hands and feet, a small-footprint high-frequency probe might be well worth the investment.

## System Features: "Bells and Whistles"

Features to look for when purchasing a system will largely be dictated by how one intends to use the system and to what extent one desires to develop expertise in musculoskeletal ultrasound.

Some systems are engineered to be more or less "plug and play." These machines have very limited ability to fine-tune images and settings. They are designed for those practitioners who simply want to turn on their machine and go to work.

For example, there are systems available that lack the ability to adjust scanning frequency independently of scanning depth. The software "assumes" that when the depth is increased, the frequency must be correspondingly decreased to image deeper structures. While this is generally the case, there are times when one may want to decrease the frequency but not the depth. For example, sometimes it is easier to see a needle when performing a guided injection by using a lower frequency, but increasing the depth would compromise the quality of the image. Conversely, it may occasionally be desirable to increase the depth without changing the frequency, such as when scanning the posterior glenohumeral joint.

The ability to adjust scanning depth varies by systems. Some machines "toggle" from one depth to the next, and you cannot go backward; you must continue to toggle forward and back around to the beginning. Likewise, some systems have limited—or no—ability to set and adjust focal points or zones. This is done automatically and determined by built-in software algorithms.

Some systems are touch screen only; they lack a true keyboard. Similar to an iPad, they use a virtual keyboard that appears on the screen.

While some units have separate time-gain compensator sliders (TGCs), others lack this feature or else have it built in to the software settings. TGCs are analogous to a graphic equalizer in a stereo system. They allow the user to adjust a particular band or portion of the image to compensate for variations in tissue density and attenuation.

There are other helpful features to consider. The ability to do side-by-side on-screen comparisons, comparing the pathological side to the "normal" side, can be useful. Beam steer technology, the ability to angle the sound beam to make it more perpendicular to the needle to help in visualization, for example, can be quite useful when performing guided injections. Panoramic view can be helpful when trying to image a structure that extends beyond the visible area of the screen, such as when trying to capture an image of the entire length of the rectus femoris muscle.

Annotation features is another area to evaluate. How easy is it to label your images on screen or to change the labels? Does the system offer the ability to create a custom "library" of commonly used terms? Some systems will use different libraries based on the particular scanning settings used, such as one library of annotation labels when scanning the foot and another library when scanning the shoulder.

Post-image processing ability is yet another feature to consider. The ability to label, to relabel, or even to change the appearance of an image or to take a measurement after the image has been taken and saved can be important. Sometimes it can be more efficient to go back and label or fine-tune your images after the visit instead of slowing down while performing the actual exam to change labels. Some systems do not allow any post-image processing at all; once the image is saved, it cannot be labeled or altered.

Finally, the ability to adjust the various parameters of power Doppler, such as pulse repetition frequency (PRF), wall filter, flash suppression, and gain, varies widely from one system to another. For those practitioners who utilize power Doppler to assess for neovascularity or synovitis or who find Doppler helpful to locate nerves via their attendant vascular structures, the ability to fine-tune Doppler settings can be an important consideration.

Oftentimes ultrasound novices are intimidated by systems that have a high degree of adjustability. For many, a less complicated "set it and forget it" system will meet their needs perfectly. As one becomes more skilled in ultrasound, however, the desire to move beyond the basics can be hampered by the limitations of certain systems. In those cases, the choice becomes one of buying a more robust system from the outset and "growing into it" or choosing a system that is more user-friendly to start and then upgrading over time.

## Warranties and Extended Service Contracts

Ultrasound systems and probes are all expensive items. True to the saying, if something can break or go wrong, it will—at least, eventually. Most new systems come with a 1-year factory warranty. Beyond that, purchasing an extended warranty is worth considering. Transducers alone can cost $5,000–10,000 to replace. In addition, most extended service contracts guarantee service within a specified period of time, often in 1–2 days. This minimizes system downtime and revenue loss. Without a service contract, you are often placed in a queue to wait for service, and repairs can be expensive.

Not all extended service contracts need to be purchased from the manufacturer nor do they need to be purchased with a new system. There are companies that specialize in selling used and demo ultrasound equipment, and many offer extended service contracts; in some cases, they offer better pricing and service than the manufacturer.

By far the most important factor when choosing a system is to pick one that will meet anticipated needs while also fitting within any budget constraints. You should demo each system you are considering by having the company sales representative bring a machine to your office for a day or two to try on a variety of patients and scanning conditions. Most companies will gladly oblige such requests.

## Transducer Care and Cleaning

Proper care and cleaning of ultrasound transducers is important, not only to maintain proper probe functioning but also to prevent infections and transmission of communicable diseases.

The official position statement of the American Institute of Ultrasound in Medicine states, "Practices must meet or exceed the quality assurance guidelines specified in Routine Quality Assurance for Diagnostic Ultrasound Equipment" [1]:

- Instrumentation used for diagnostic testing must be maintained in good operating condition and undergo routine calibration at least once a year.
- All ultrasound equipment must be serviced at least annually, according to the manufacturers' specifications or more frequently if problems arise.
- There must be routine inspection and testing for electrical safety of all existing equipment.

Most ultrasound manufacturers offer guidelines for cleaning and maintaining the transducer. Practitioners are advised to follow the specific manufacturer's guidelines to prevent voiding any warranties. However, many guidelines are more general.

A generic cleaning protocol may include these points:

- Clean the transducer after each use (follow the manufacturer's guidelines).
- For the most part, the transducer is going to be used on the skin and is not going to be exposed to blood or any other bodily fluids. Wiping the transducer off with a soft cloth using a mild soap and water is acceptable after each use.
- An alternative to this is to clean the transducer with antimicrobial/germicidal wipes, with low alcohol content, such as PDI's Sani-Cloth (www.pdipdi.com/healthcare/surface_disinfect.aspx), a soft disposable cloth dampened

with CaviCide (http://metrex2.reachlocal.net/), or something similar.

- Before proceeding with any sterile procedure (injection or placing transducer near an open wound or lesion on the dermis), the transducer should be cleaned using an antimicrobial wipe. Many practitioners use sterile sheaths, so the transducer is never directly exposed to bodily fluids. If this is not the case, care should be taken to not expose the transducer directly to bodily fluids. If this happens, follow manufacturer's guidelines to properly sanitize the transducer.

The following should also be considered to properly maintain the transducer:

- It is always a good idea to reference the owner's manual or directly contact the company before using any non-referenced cleaner or sterilization techniques, so the transducer is not damaged.
- Avoid direct contact of the transducer head and cable with sharp objects, such as needles or scalpels.
- Do not clean the transducer with a brush or sponge without consulting the manufacturer, because these objects may damage the transducer head.
- When cleaning or disinfecting the transducer cable, always elevate the head above the cable. This insures that the liquid on the cable does not drip onto the transducer head.
- Train all office staff with a written protocol/checklist for cleaning and maintenance of the ultrasound equipment.

## Summary

Choosing an ultrasound system involves consideration of a number of important variables, only one of which should be price. Intended use, the degree of desire of the physician to master ultrasound, and physical space limitations are also important factors. Almost all of the current ultrasound systems marketed toward the musculoskeletal market will do an adequate job for the majority of musculoskeletal work. However, as the saying goes, the "Devil's in the details," and it behooves the physician to at least consider some of those details outlined in this chapter. Price should actually be among the least of the factors considered. In the vast majority of cases, over time, your ultrasound system will more than pay for itself. And over the course of 3–5 years (the length of time most practices keep a system before upgrading), a few thousand dollars become much less significant than the benefits of having a system that not only meets your needs but also one that is a joy and satisfaction to use.

## Reference

1. http://www.aium.org/publications/viewStatement.aspx?id=26.

# Knobology

## Allyson S. Howe

## The Machine

A review of two commonly used control panels on ultrasound machines from SonoSite and GE (General Electric) is included here for the purpose of demonstration. The principles of image capturing and quality improvement of images should be similar regardless of the brand of machine that you are using, although the specific terms for such functions may be different.

## Mode

There are various types (modes) of ultrasound images that are commonly obtained.

In B-mode (brightness mode) ultrasound, a linear array of transducers about the width of a credit card simultaneously scans a plane through the body that can be viewed as a two-dimensional image on screen. This is sometimes described as 2D mode, and it provides the single still images that are frequently used for documentation purposes to define structures.

M-mode (motion mode) is used to capture multiple images in sequence. In simple terms, it collects a video of a particular scan.

## Doppler Mode

The Doppler effect is used to help define the presence, direction, and velocity of blood flow. It is useful and can be used in combination to help provide adequate information about the blood flow around a particular anatomical area.

## Color Flow (GE) and Color (SonoSite)

The use of color to define blood flow is a useful feature. Superimposed on a grayscale ultrasound image, the use of color flow helps determine whether blood flow exists (i.e., identifies location of blood vessels) and is conventionally set up to show blue color when the blood flows away from the transducer and red color when it flows towards it. Flow velocity cannot be measured within this feature.

### Clinical Application

When performing a joint injection—of the hip joint, for example—the use of color Doppler can identify the location of blood vessels so that the angle of approach can be set to avoid the path of the vessel.

## Pulsed Wave (GE) and Doppler (SonoSite)

This provides an image of a moving object along with its waveform. It can give you the presence of flow as well as define the velocity of blood flow within a vessel.

### Clinical Application

During echocardiograms, it can define the velocity of flow across a heart valve.

## Power Doppler

This is color Doppler mode with high sensitivity to blood flow such that many small vessels are visible. Vessels that are small or that have very slow flow rates can be seen using this technique. The weakness in using this technique lies in its high sensitivity; it can create an artifact in certain situations, misidentifying vessels that are not there. This typically appears as a dense area of "color" on the screen and is generally due to unintended operator movement of the transducer/probe and will resolve quickly with a steady hand. Additionally, it does not tell directionality or velocity of the flow seen.

### Clinical Application

Power Doppler can be used to evaluate neovascularization in the setting of chronic tendinosis.

A.S. Howe, M.D. (✉)
Department of Family Medicine, Maine Medical Center, 272 Congress Street, Portland, ME 04101, USA
e-mail: howea1@mmc.org

J.M. Daniels and W.W. Dexter (eds.), *Basics of Musculoskeletal Ultrasound*, DOI 10.1007/978-1-4614-3215-9_4, © Springer Science+Business Media New York 2013

## Frequency

A transducer has an inherent ability to send a range of sound wave frequencies towards tissue that are described by the unit's megahertz (MHz). The higher the frequency of waves being sent, the higher the resolution of the image will be. However, higher-frequency waves are unable to penetrate deeply in tissue and will be unable to clearly visualize deep structures; this is the cost of using a high-frequency probe. Low-frequency probes are able to penetrate in tissue to find deeper structures but at the cost of a lower-resolution image.

## Image Balance

### Gain

Changing the gain is analogous to amplifying or suppressing the volume of signal in an image. By adjusting the gain up or down, you may find it easier to visualize certain structures. Each ultrasound machine is equipped with an "autogain," which is the machine's interpretation of the optimal level of gain for the body part or structure being scanned. When first starting out with scanning, the use of autogain is likely going to be a useful tool. We recommend adjusting the gain manually to affect the image quality, then comparing it to the autogain for image improvement.

### Time-Gained Compensation

The sound waves emitted by your transducer at the surface of the skin will attenuate as they travel through tissue on their way to your target. The time-gained compensation (TGC) set of controls help you to fine-tune the gain in the areas of interest on the screen for improved visualization of the structures you are intending to view.

### Depth

The depth to which a sound wave can penetrate tissue is linked with the frequency capability within your transducer. As noted previously, a high-frequency probe will provide high-quality images at a low depth, whereas a low-frequency probe will excel at giving deeper structure images, though there may be a compromise in image clarity. When first starting an ultrasound examination, adjustment of the depth of the picture is key to ensure that the structures you are evaluating can be seen within the field of view. On the right side of the monitor, there will be a measurement expressing (often in centimeters) the depth of penetration the probe is set for and how deep within the tissue your structure is.

### Clinical Application

Depth is very helpful in situations in which you are intending to make an ultrasound-guided injection and need to determine the proper position and length of the needle you'll need to use to reach a particular structure.

## Focal Zones

In order to visualize fine anatomy (i.e., follow a nerve course) or to just focus the beam on a particular narrow anatomical region, the use of focal zones can be very helpful. On the GE model machines, there is a focal zone dial to help adjust this setting. This same effect on a SonoSite machine is accomplished with near and far gain.

### Clinical Application

Placing the object of interest into a focal zone ensures a higher-quality picture of that object for identification and also for a clearer injection visualization, as may occur with a calcific tendinopathy injection, for example, where you would choose to put the calcific density in the focal zone for clarity.

## Documenting the Examination

### Text

Labeling an ultrasound image with text is an important step in documenting your examination for the medical record. The first step in documenting is finding the image you are intending to visualize and freezing the frame at that spot. On a SonoSite machine, choosing "Text" will provide you with a cursor on the screen. The cursor position can be changed by moving it around using the key pad. After you have added the desired text, choose "Freeze" and "Save" to keep the image for documentation. When you choose "Freeze" again to unfreeze the frame, the text will remain present. This is helpful if you are taking different views of the same structure. If you need to remove the text, you'll choose "Delete" and continue scanning.

On GE models, after freezing the screen, you can begin typing on the keyboard, and text will show up on the screen where the cursor left off or in the left upper corner. That text can be moved to the location you prefer by rolling the rollerball into position.

### Clinical Application

It will be necessary to label images with text to clarify structures for documentation and for the purpose of orientation, such as labeling "left" and "right."

### Measurements

There will be many times when a measurement of a particular object seen on a screen is important. Using the freeze button, it is important to first freeze the frame of the picture of the object you are trying to measure. Using a SonoSite machine, choosing "Caliper" will provide you with a moveable measuring device. Adjust the first portion of the cursor by moving your finger on the key pad. Now align that cursor with the left end of the object. Choose "Select." You will now have access to the opposite cursor and can set this up to measure the right side of the object. If the object you are measuring is elliptical, choose "Ellipse" function at the left lower side of the keyboard, and an adjustable ellipse will form.

## Clinical Application

You will find it helpful to measure linear objects such as the length of a tear as well as elliptical or circular objects such as the size of an abscess or a cyst prior to drainage.

## Initial Steps

Setting up your machine prior to scanning is important to get the highest-quality picture possible. This includes choosing any presets that may be available on your machine (i.e., choose the body part you are intending to view, and ensure you are in musculoskeletal imaging preset). Adding the patient's name and identifying information (i.e., date of birth) is an important initial step for documenting the examination. Ensure the transducer you wish to use is connected to the machine. You can predict somewhat which transducer you need to use by considering the depth of the object you are intending to study (i.e., the carpal tunnel is very shallow, the hip joint is very deep) and the size of the object you wish to study (i.e., it will be easier to use a small probe for fingers, larger probe for the shoulder).

As you begin your scanning of a particular body part, the first adjustment you may need to make is with depth. Adjust the depth of your image until the body part of interest can be seen in the field of view.

Next, adjust your focal zone. On some ultrasound machines, the focal zone can be adjusted to a specific location within the field. On other machines, you will adjust either the superficial or deeper zone, depending on where the object you are visualizing lies.

Next, adjust the gain on the screen. By adjusting the gain (i.e., whiteness or darkness), you will see that with increased or decreased contrast, certain structures come into better view.

Remember that you may need to readjust the settings on the screen as you scan through for different views of anatomical structures.

## Clinical Exercise

1. Become very familiar with the controls on the machine by doing the following:
   - Demonstrate that you can easily change transducers.
   - Label scan for patient's name, date of birth, date of scan, and body part.
   - Adjust the depth of the field so the image takes up the whole screen.
   - If your machine has presets for different tissues or body parts, please do this.
   - If your machine has focal zones, adjust those to the area that you want to scan.
   - Adjust the gain on the machine in two extremes—one bright and one dark.
2. Record a scanned image—one bright and one dark—with the above settings and patient identification. Practice to the point that this is "second nature" by holding the probe in one hand and adjusting the settings in the other. Save these two images for documentation/homework.
3. Repeat the above process, but this time, record an image with:
   - Caliper measurements of a structure on the scan. Measure length, width, and circumference of structure of a muscle, tendon, or nerve.
   - Perform a dynamic scan, such as impingement exam of the shoulder or valgus stressing of the ulnar collateral ligament of the thumb or elbow.
   - Turn on color Doppler and identify an artery and vein.
   - If your machine has the capability, perform a panoramic exam of a structure such as the Achilles or patellar tendon.

## Suggested Reading

Bianchi S, Martinoli C. Ultrasound of the musculoskeletal system. New York City, NY: Springer; 2007.

Jacobson JA. Fundamentals of musculoskeletal ultrasound. Philadelphia, PA: Saunders/Elsevier; 2007.

McNally E. Practical musculoskeletal ultrasound. Philadelphia, PA: Elsevier; 2007.

Stoller DW. Stoller's atlas of orthopaedics and sports medicine. Baltimore, MD: Lippincott Williams & Wilkins; 2008.

European Society of Musculoskeletal Radiology. http://www.essr.org/cms/website.php?id=/en/essr_home.htm

# Tissue Scanning

**5**

## J. Herbert Stevenson

## Ultrasound Equipment

The ultrasound equipment at its most basic level includes a transducer (probe) connected to an ultrasound computer that includes a CPU, monitor, keyboard, transducer controls, disk drive, and often a printer (Fig. 5.1). The transducer contains quartz crystals that utilize the piezoelectric electric effect, which transforms electrical current into sound waves and vice versa. The piezoelectric effect allows the probe to generate sound waves that propagate through soft tissue. The sound waves are able to be reflected back or echo at varying rates depending upon the type of tissue they encounter. The probe is then able to receive the mechanical sound waves and transform them into an electric current that can be analyzed by the CPU. The data are subsequently displayed as two-dimensional real-time images on the screen.

Probes come in different shapes and sizes (Fig. 5.2) depending upon the clinical indication. A linear probe is most often utilized in musculoskeletal medicine. A linear probe allows for more accurate evaluation of structures close to the skin surface compared with a curvilinear probe that allows great resolution of deeper structures. Linear probes transmit at a higher frequency, generally in the range of 8–18 MHz. The higher frequency allows them to obtain greater resolution of near-field structures at the sacrifice of depth and penetration. When greater depth of visualization is required, a curvilinear probe is preferred. Common clinical indications in musculoskeletal ultrasound for utilization of a curvilinear probe include ultrasound of the hip, spine, and glenohumeral joint.

J.H. Stevenson, M.D. (✉)
Department of Family and Community Medicine, University of Massachusetts Medical Center, University of Massachusetts Medical School, 281 Lincoln Street, Worcester, MA 01605, USA

Department of Orthopedics and Rehabilitation, University of Massachusetts Medical Center, University of Massachusetts Medical School, 281 Lincoln Street, Worcester, MA 01605, USA
e-mail: John.Stevenson@umassmemorial.org

Ultrasound of small structures, including the hands and feet, may be best visualized with a small-footprint ("hockey stick") probe.

## Anatomic Terminology

A sound understanding of body sections and anatomical planes is required in order to properly perform and interpret musculoskeletal ultrasound. Body sections can be divided into the sagittal, transverse, and coronal planes (Fig. 5.3). A sagittal plane is a vertical plane passing from front to back through the body separating it into a left and right partition. A transverse plane is one that passes along a horizontal plane dividing the body into an upper and lower partition. A coronal plane is a vertical plane passing from side to side that divides the body into ventral and dorsal partitions.

Anatomic definitions illustrated in Fig. 5.3 include anterior, posterior, proximal, distal, lateral, medial, cranial, and caudal.

## Ultrasound Terminology

Ultrasound terminology differs from descriptive terminology utilized in other modalities such as MRI because it describes the echogenicity of the structures being imaged. Echogenicity refers to the extent to which different substances and structures within the body reflect sound waves. The greater the percentage of sound waves that are reflected from a particular structure, the higher the echogenicity of the structure detected by the probe. Different tissue types will produce unique echogenic images that tend to be consistent across tissue types (i.e., muscle, tendon, bone). The higher a structure's echogenicity, the brighter it will be displayed on the monitor. Conversely, the lower a structure's echogenicity, the darker it will appear. The following is a list of descriptive ultrasound terminology:

- Hyperechoic: high reflectivity displayed as a bright or light signal. Bone and tendon are examples of hyperechoic

J.M. Daniels and W.W. Dexter (eds.), *Basics of Musculoskeletal Ultrasound*, DOI 10.1007/978-1-4614-3215-9_5, © Springer Science+Business Media New York 2013

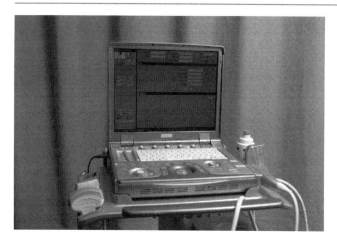

**Fig. 5.1** Image of ultrasound equipment

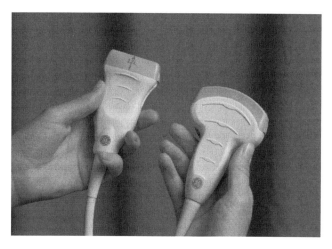

**Fig. 5.2** Linear, curvilinear, and "hockey stick" probe

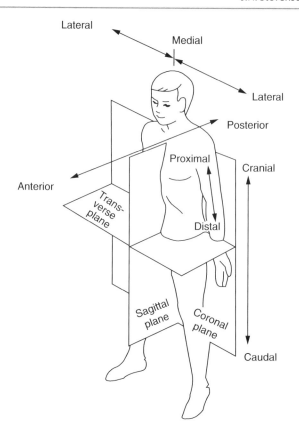

**Fig. 5.3** Sagittal, transverse, and coronal planes. Anterior, posterior, proximal, distal, lateral, medial, cranial, and caudal. Adapted from http://msis.jsc.nasa.gov/images/Section03/Image64.gif

objects (Fig. 5.4a: note hyperechoic acromion [with acoustic shadowing] and humerus).

- Isoechoic: when two adjacent objects are of equal echogenicity (Fig. 5.4b: note quadriceps tendon, three bands, hard to distinguish [isoechoic]).
- Hypoechoic: low reflectivity displayed as a darker area. Muscle fiber bundles are an example of hypoechoic structures (Fig. 5.4c: muscle fibers of gastrocnemius and soleus muscles).
- Anechoic: absence of ultrasound reflectivity/signal displayed as a black area. Fluid is commonly displayed as anechoic (Fig. 5.4d: short-axis view of median nerve [MN] and anechoic ulnar artery [UA]).

## Technical Aspects of Ultrasound Image Acquisition

The ability to acquire a clear and accurate image with musculoskeletal ultrasound requires a systematic approach along with a sound understanding of three-dimensional anatomy. Additionally, the ability to manipulate the probe in its three planes of movement is crucial, as even slight alterations in probe position will significantly affect the quality of the image. Ultrasound competency requires routine practice and repetition to become proficient in its use.

## Probe Handling

Probe handling is essential to the proper performance of an accurate and repeatable ultrasound exam. A steady and secure handling of the probe will facilitate a clear image with minimal artifact. The probe should be held in a steady but not rigid grip between the thumb on one side of the probe and the second and third fingers on the other side. The fourth and fifth fingers, along with ulnar/hypothenar aspect of the palm, should rest on the skin of the patient examined. This connection to the patient at all times will facilitate a secure platform from which to manipulate the probe for optimal image resolution (Fig. 5.5a, b).

## Probe Coupling Agents

Coupling of the probe to the skin is necessary to provide a link between the transducer and the patient. The sound waves produced and received by the transducer will not pass through air. A coupling agent is required and generally consists of a gel or standoff pad.

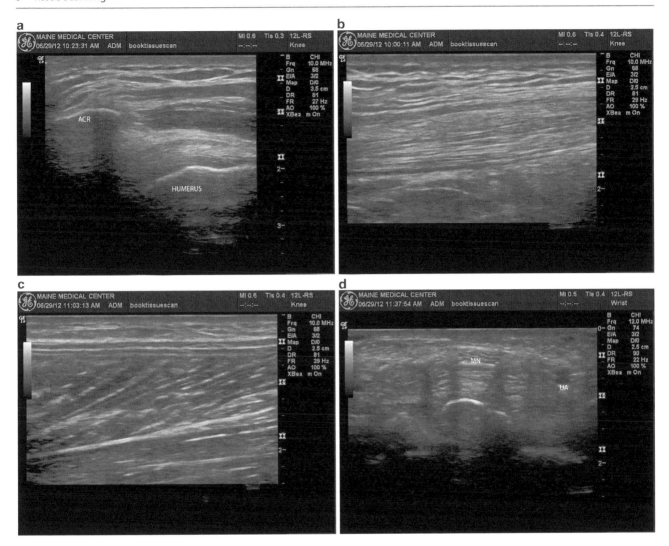

**Fig. 5.4** (**a–d**) Examples of hyperechoic, isoechoic, hypoechoic, and anechoic

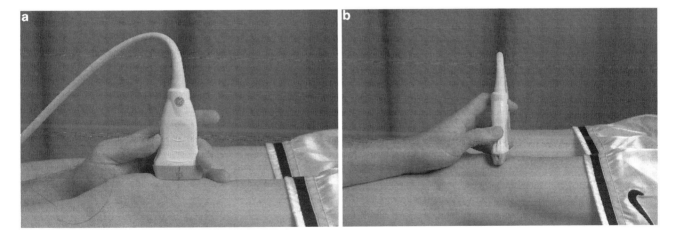

**Fig. 5.5** (**a, b**) Proper handling of an ultrasound probe

## Gel

Ultrasound gel is an ideal medium that allows for coupling of the ultrasound signal without providing distortion. Gel should completely cover the probe surface but not be too excessive so as to cause one to lose one's grip of the probe. Bony surfaces or irregular surfaces may require additional gel to compensate for the peaks and valleys of the surface, allowing for uniform coupling. Finally, sterile gel should be utilized for ultrasound-guided injections/aspirations/needle procedures when the needle may potentially come in contact with the gel.

## Standoff Pad

The standoff pad is made of an acoustically transparent medium that provides a compliant surface to image bony/uneven surfaces. Standoff pads also assist in imaging shallow or sensitive areas by increasing the depth of the structures and providing a cushioned surface (Fig. 5.6).

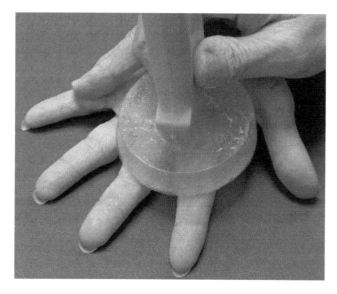

**Fig. 5.6** Standoff pad

## Probe Orientation to the Patient

In order to maintain consistency, the left side of the probe should correlate with the left side of the screen, while the right side of the probe should correlate with the right side of the screen. Most commercial probes will have a notch or indicator light on one side of the probe that aligns with the same side of the display, allowing for rapid detection of orientation. An important point is to ensure that both the examiner and the patient are comfortable during the procedure. The patient may be positioned on a table, recliner, or stool. The examiner should be sitting with the US monitor close and at the proper height (eye level) to comfortably perform the exam.

By convention, the probe should be orientated cephalad when in a sagittal or coronal plane. When the transducer is in the axial plane, the left side of the probe should align with the right side of the patient's body; conversely, the right side of the probe should align with the left side of the patient's body. Some clinicians may reverse this depending on their hand dominance during certain procedures. A simple way to check for probe orientation related to the patient and the screen is to gently tap one side of the probe (with gel applied) with a finger and look at the screen to determine probe orientation. Any orientation is acceptable as long as it is marked and documented.

## Probe Axis to the Imaged Structure

Once the probe is placed on the skin, the probe will need to align with the long or short axis to the structure one is visualizing. The long (or longitudinal) axis is along the plane that parallels the greatest length of the structure, while the short (or transverse) axis runs perpendicular to the long axis and parallel to the greatest width of the structure (Fig. 5.7a, b). Figure 5.7a is an ultrasound screenshot corresponding to the long-axis probe placement over the quadriceps tendon

a
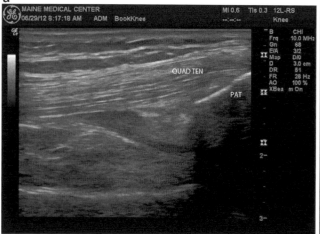

b
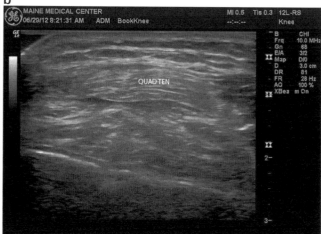

**Fig. 5.7** (**a**, **b**) Long- and short-axis views

demonstrated in Fig. 5.5a. Figure 5.7b is an ultrasound screenshot corresponding to the transverse probe placement over the quadriceps tendon demonstrated in Fig. 5.5b.

## Probe Manipulations

Once on the skin, the ultrasound probe can be manipulated along any of its three axes of movement ($X$, $Y$, $Z$ axis) to facilitate proper image acquisition. Key to image acquisition is the centering of the object desired and optimizing the

ultrasound probe, so the beam is aimed perpendicular to the structure. The manipulation of the probe is particularly important when imaging curved or irregular structures. The five probe planes of manipulation as defined by the American Institute of Ultrasound in Medicine are listed below:

- *Sliding*: translates the probe along the length or width to the structures without rocking or tilting the probe. This allows visualization of the structure in length as well as width (Fig. 5.8a, b).
- *Rocking*: tilting (heel-toe movement) of the probe to one edge or the other (Fig. 5.8c, d). This is helpful when there

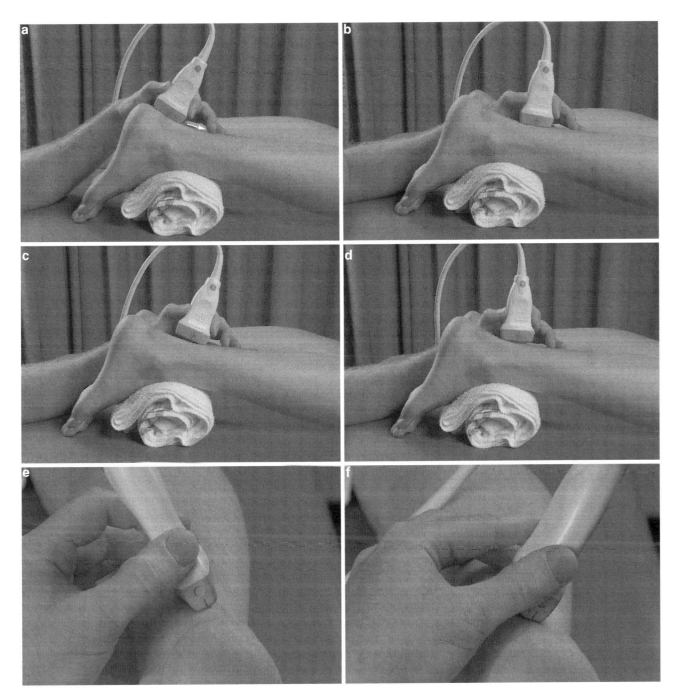

**Fig. 5.8** (**a–i**) Example of five probe movements: sliding, rocking, tilting, rotating, compression

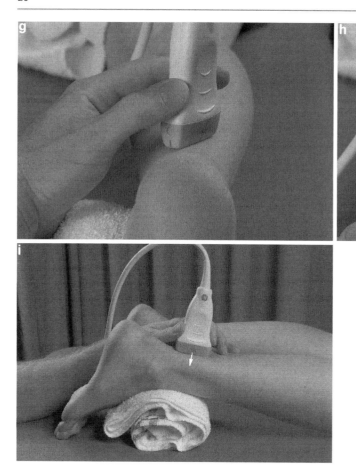

**Fig. 5.8** (continued)

is a narrow window of imaging, and adjacent structures are to be centered or visualized. Rocking may also facilitate extending the field of view, such as in the cephalic or caudal direction. A common example of rocking is utilized to visualize the proximal biceps tendon that runs in a deep to superficial direction as it passes through the bicipital groove.

- *Tilting*: the side-to-side movement of the probe to bring additional planes of tissue into focus without sliding the probe (Fig. 5.8e, f).
- *Rotating*: movement of the probe in clockwise or counterclockwise movement. Rotating facilitates obtaining the long- and short-axis views of structures (Fig. 5.8g, h).
- *Compression*: pressing down with the probe. Compressible structures such as veins or bursa fluid will decrease or disappear with compression. Compression also allows deeper structures to appear more superficial. Finally, compression may allow proper contact between the probe and patient to allow clear visualization on curved or irregular structures (Fig. 5.8i).

## Focusing/Knobology

Focusing may be done prior to placing the probe on the skin if the ultrasound machine has appropriate presets for the structures imaged (i.e., shoulder, knee, wrist). Conversely, focusing may occur manually after the probe has been placed on the skin. A thorough understanding of the controls and their appropriate settings ("knobology") is another key element in obtaining an accurate and optimal image. Knobology is discussed in detail in Chap. 4.

## Ultrasound Imaging Artifact

Numerous ultrasound artifacts can occur and affect the proper imaging and interpretation of anatomic structures. These often occur due to the change of sound propagation through different tissue densities as well as alterations in the path taken by the US beam. An understanding of these artifacts and why they occur will enhance one's ability to properly interpret ultrasound images.

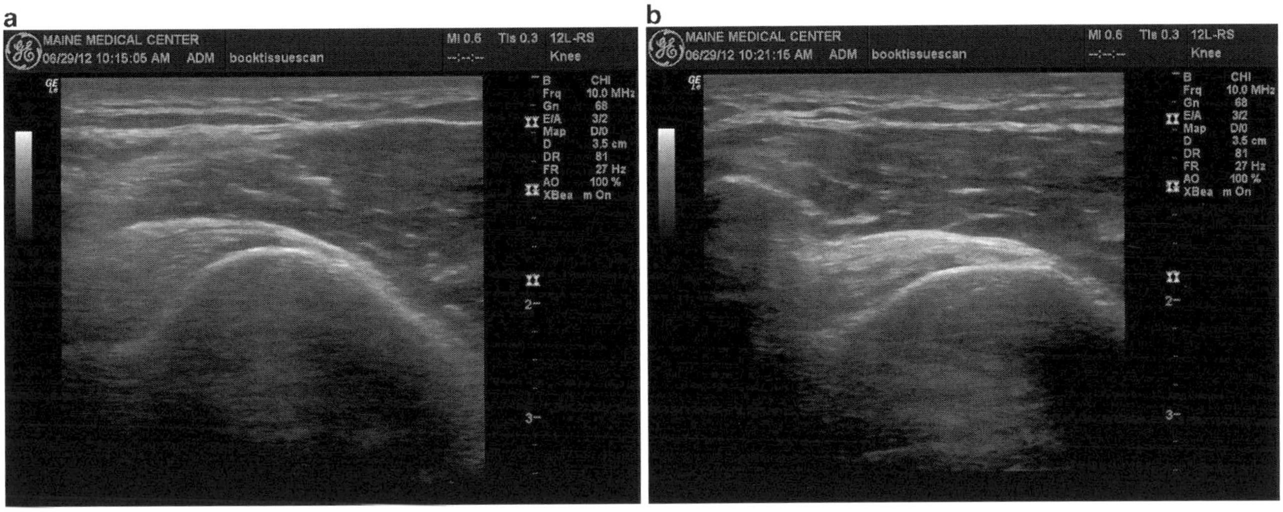

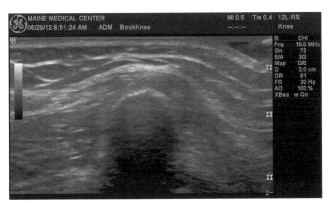

**Fig. 5.9** (**a**, **b**) Example of anisotropy

**Fig. 5.10** Example of acoustic shadowing

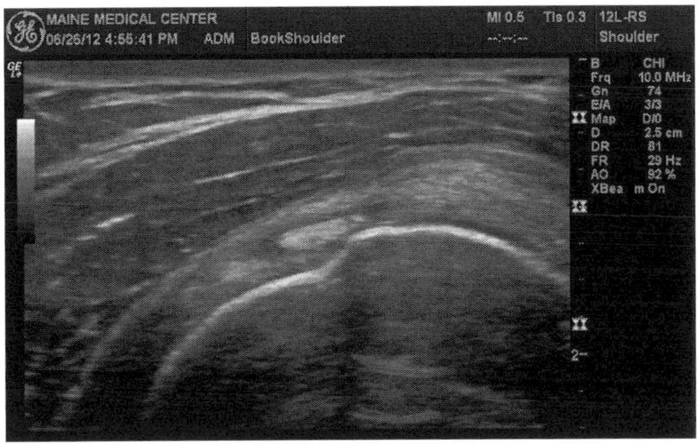

**Fig. 5.11** Example of acoustic enhancement

## Anisotropy

Anisotropy is the property of tendons, nerves, and muscle to display a different appearance depending upon the angle the ultrasound signal is directed (insonation). When an ultrasound sound beam is at an angle less than 85°, the majority of the sound waves will not reflect back to the transducer. This results in a normally hyperechoic (bright) structure appearing hypoechoic (dark). Tendons exhibit the greatest amount of anisotropy, and the loss of the normal tendon fibrillar structure may be misinterpreted as a tear or area of tendinosis. The operator can correct the anisotropy by angling the probe sound waves perpendicular to the structure with a rocking (heel-toe) maneuver. Figure 5.9a shows anisotropy on rotator cuff, and Fig. 5.9b shows anisotropy resolved using heel-toe rocking.

## Acoustic Shadowing

Acoustic shadowing is the attenuation of sound waves due to very dense substance that reflects nearly all the sound waves. Figure 5.10 shows acoustic shadowing on the patella.

This results in a lack of visualization deep to the structure. Commonly, this can occur from bone, foreign bodies, and intratendinous/muscular calcifications.

## Acoustic Enhancement

Acoustic enhancement results from sound waves passing through anechoic (black appearing) structures (fluid). The structures deep to the fluid then appear more echogenic than the same tissue on either side of the fluid. Figure 5.11 shows acoustic enhancement of the biceps tendon.

## Reverberation Artifact

Reverberation artifact results from sound waves reflecting back and forth between the surface of the transducer and a highly echogenic structure. The resulting image is one of evenly spaced lines of the structure at increasing depths. Needle guidance is a common scenario in which reverberation artifact can occur when the needle is near perpendicular

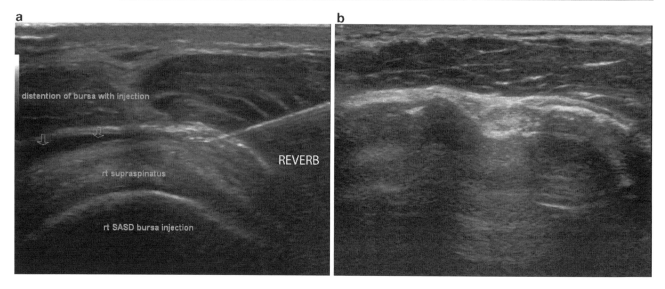

**Fig. 5.12** (**a**, **b**) Example of reverberation artifact and comet tail artifact

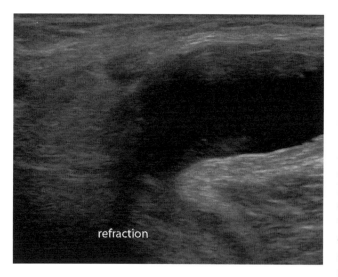

**Fig. 5.13** Example of refraction artifact

to the probe (Fig. 5.12a). The *comet tail artifact* is a form of reverberation artifact that can be seen with an object that strongly reflects the ultrasound waves, such as crystals and metallic and glass foreign bodies. The reverberation signal is seen deep to the structure in gradually decreasing size, similar in appearance to a comet tail (Fig. 5.12b).

## Refraction Artifact

Refraction artifact is also known as edge shadowing and occurs distal to the edges of curvilinear structures. Sound waves impacting a curved surface are refracted/bent from their original direction, resulting in falsely hypoechoic edge shadowing distally (Fig. 5.13).

## Ultrasound Imaging of Normal Tissue

The understanding and identification of normal tissue architecture is fundamental to performing musculoskeletal ultrasound. The following is a brief overview of the different tissue characteristics that help differentiate one from the other.

### Skeletal Muscle

Skeletal muscle is viewed as a heterogeneous structure with hypoechoic muscle fiber bundles interspersed with hyperechoic stromal connective tissue (perimysium). On long-axis view, this will give a pennate appearance similar to barbs converging on a feather (Fig. 5.14a, gastrocnemius and soleus muscles, long axis). The hyperechoic stromal connective tissue will converge towards the end of the muscle into the muscle tendon. Muscle on cross-section is displayed as a "starry night" appearance, with wavy, hyperechoic connective tissue interspersed with the hypoechoic muscle fibers (Fig. 5.14b, gastrocnemius and soleus muscles, short axis).

### Tendons

Tendons are displayed as a mixture of bright echogenic tendon fibers interspersed with hypoechoic surrounding connective tissue in a parallel course. On long-axis view, this results in a linear fibrillar appearance. Tendons imaged on short-axis view will demonstrate hyperechoic collagen bundles seen in short-axis view interspersed between hypoechoic connective tissue. Because of the compact fibrillar structure of tendons, they can suffer from anisotropy artifact if visualized at an angle less than perpendicular (Fig. 5.15a, Achilles tendon in long axis; Fig. 5.15b, Achilles tendon in short axis).

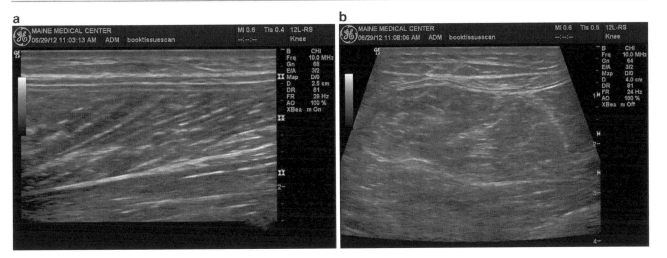

**Fig. 5.14** (**a, b**) Example of skeletal muscle, long and short axis

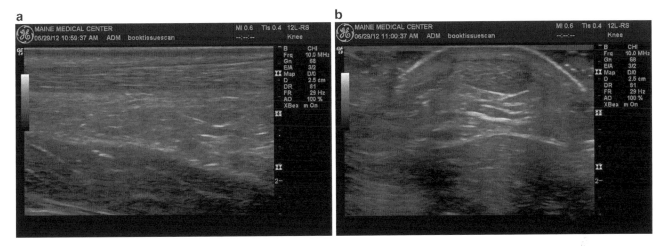

**Fig. 5.15** (**a, b**) Example of tendon, long and short axis

## Ligaments

Ligaments are visualized as bright hyperechoic linear fibrils with linear areas of hypoechoic connective tissue (Fig. 5.16). Ligaments have a similar appearance to tendons but tend to be more compact, with their individual collagen fibrils more closely aligned. Ligaments may also suffer from anisotropy artifact when imaged.

## Fascia

Fascia is displayed as hyperechoic (bright) structure (Fig. 5.17, fascia in hamstring). Fascia thickness can vary depending on the structure and location imaged.

## Subcutaneous Tissue

Subcutaneous tissue will be displayed as a hyperechoic (bright) superficial structure (epidermis and dermis). Deep to this will be the subcutaneous fat displayed as a hypoechoic

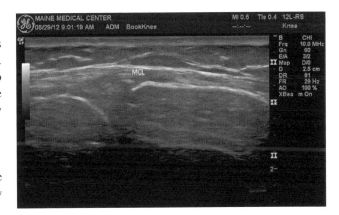

**Fig. 5.16** Example of ligament

(dark) adipose tissue irregularly interspersed with hyperechoic connective tissue (Fig. 5.18, subcutaneous tissue over medial gastrocnemius).

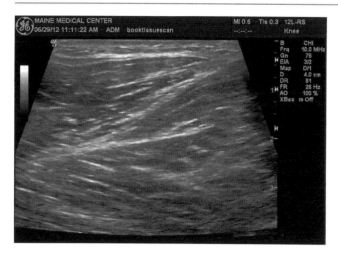

**Fig. 5.17** Example of fascia

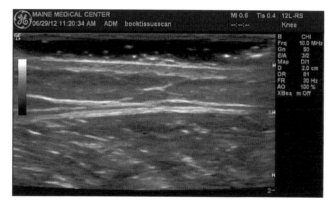

**Fig. 5.18** Example of subcutaneous tissue

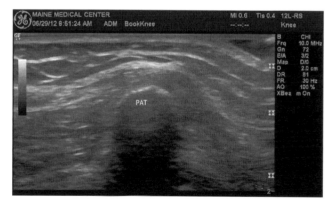

**Fig. 5.19** Example of cortical bone

## Cortical Bone

Cortical bone is shown as hyperechoic (bright) linear line with posterior acoustic shadowing due to complete reflection of the ultrasound beam (Fig. 5.19, transverse view of hyperechoic patella with acoustic shadowing).

## Peripheral Nerves

Peripheral nerves are displayed as larger hypoechoic nerve fascicles embedded within smaller hyperechoic interfascicular epineurium. Peripheral nerves visualized on short-axis view will display the characteristic "honeycomb" appearance. On long-axis view, they will be displayed as a "train track" structure (Fig. 5.20a, median nerve, short axis; Fig. 5.20b, median nerve, long axis).

## Bursa

Bursa that is not inflamed will be seen as a small strip of anechoic (black) structure surrounded by hyperechoic (bright) peribursal fat (Fig. 5.21). When distended, it will have a larger area of anechoic or hypoechoic (dark) signal and may be filled with septations and synovial debris.

## Articular Cartilage

Articular cartilage is seen as an anechoic (black) layer overlying the periosteum (Fig. 5.22, femoral trochlear cartilage).

## Advanced Ultrasound Techniques

A fundamental advantage of ultrasound is the dynamic nature of the exam where images are obtained in real time. This allows for many advantages over static imaging techniques such as plain radiographs, CT, and MRI. The interaction between examiner, probe, and patient can greatly facilitate a dynamic exam that will allow for additional diagnostic information.

## Sono-Palpation

Sono-palpation describes the interplay between the pressure applied by the transducer and the pain perceived by the patient. This allows correlating areas of tenderness with underlying pathology.

Sono-palpation can also involve the dynamic palpation of structures to view whether they are solid or fluid filled. Solid structures will maintain their shape while filled with fluid; structures such as an effusion or bursa will compress and even disappear with compression (Fig. 5.23a, olecranon bursa with minimal compression [note debris in bursa]; Fig. 5.23b, same olecranon bursa with more compression).

## Stress Views

Stress views describe the ability to image an area while dynamically providing a stress to the structure. Examples include imaging of the ulnar collateral's anterior band while providing a valgus stress to the elbow. The integrity of the ligament can

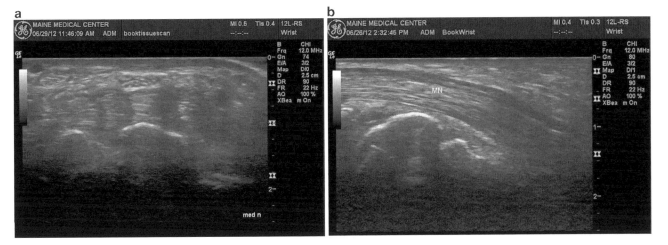

**Fig. 5.20** Example of peripheral nerves, short (**a**) and long (**b**) axis

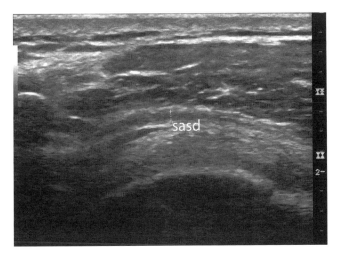

**Fig. 5.21** Example of bursa

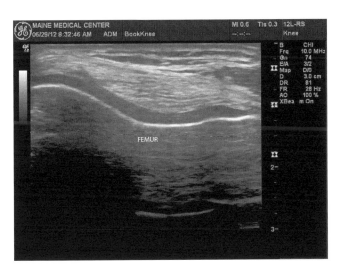

**Fig. 5.22** Example of articular cartilage

be viewed in real time as well as the amount of joint-space widening with a valgus stress (Fig. 5.24a, stress view, medial elbow, UCL tear, affected side [note gapping of joint]; Fig. 5.24b stress view, medial elbow, and unaffected side).

## Dynamic Views

Dynamic views describe the ability to image structures while moving the affected region/joint through an active or passive range of motion. An example includes watching for signs of rotator cuff/bursa impingement while passively abducting the shoulder under real-time ultrasound imaging (Fig. 5.25). Another example is having the patient actively contract an injured muscle to look for muscle widening consistent with a tear.

## Split-Screen Comparison

Split-screen comparison allows for the rapid capture of comparison views on ultrasound imaging between affected and unaffected sides of the body. The views may be saved as an image on one half of the screen with a comparison view saved to the other half. This allows for rapid comparison and analysis including measurements. The ability to easily perform comparison views is an important differentiator with MRI imaging.

## Clinical Exercise

1. Demonstrate the proper technique to scan a body part using each transducer that your machine has. Make sure that you "anchor" the probe using your fourth and fifth finger. Repeat this using both your right and left hand.

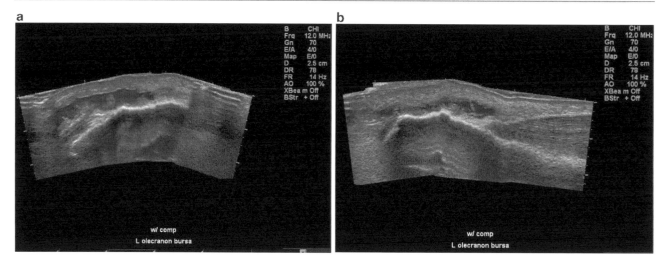

**Fig. 5.23** (**a**, **b**) Bursa, without and with probe compression

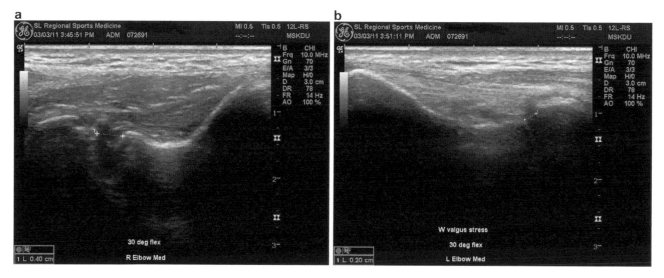

**Fig. 5.24** (**a**, **b**) Stress view of the ulna collateral ligament demonstrating joint-space widening

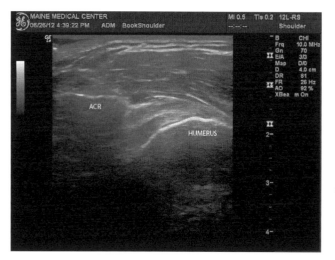

**Fig. 5.25** Dynamic US impingement test

2. Demonstrate or describe how you would position yourself, the patient, and the ultrasound machine to scan a shoulder, wrist, knee, and hip.

3. Demonstrate and, if possible, record an image while doing the following probe manipulations:
   - Sliding
   - Rocking
   - Tilting
   - Rotating
   - Compressing

4. Identify and record an image of the following (when recording the image include long- and short-axis views; also adjust gain and depth and manipulate the probe to show anisotropy where applicable):
   - Muscle
   - Tendon

- Nerve
- Ligament
- Bone
- Bursa
- Articular cartilage

5. Please obtain a large chicken breast or turkey breast. It is acceptable to leave the breast on the carcass or remove it on the underside of the breast (leave "skin side" intact). Bury in the breast (1) grape, (2) needle, (3) and one of the small bones from the carcass. If possible, place these objects at different depths.

  - Identify these objects (it is best to have someone else insert the above items, so the scanner is unaware of where the objects are).
  - Demonstrate acoustic shadowing, acoustic enhancement, reverberation artifact, refraction artifact, and sono-palpation.

- The breast can be saved and used for other clinical exercises (see Chapter on Injection Techniques).

## Suggested Reading

Harmon KG, O'Connor FG. Musculoskeletal ultrasound: taking sports medicine to the next level. Br J Sports Med. 2010;44(16):1135–6.

McNally EG. The development and clinical applications of musculoskeletal ultrasound. Skeletal Radiol. 2011;40:1223–31.

Pinzon EG, Moore RE. Musculoskeletal ultrasound. A brief overview of diagnostic and therapeutic applications in musculoskeletal medicine. Pract Pain Manag. 2009;1:34–43.

Smith J, Finnoff JT. Diagnostic and interventional musculoskeletal ultrasound: part 1. Fundamentals. PM R. 2009a;1(1):64–75.

Smith J, Finnoff JT. Diagnostic and interventional musculoskeletal ultrasound: part 2. Clinical applications. PM R. 2009b;1(2):162–77.

# Hand and Fingers

Matthew C. Bayes

## Approach to the Joint

The hand and fingers have a complex anatomic design to maximize movement and dexterity. Taken together they are comprised of 14 phalanges and 5 metacarpal bones. The volar aspect of the fingers includes two flexor tendons: the flexor digitorum superficialis and flexor digitorum profundus. The profundus lies deep and inserts on the proximal aspect of the distal phalanx, while the superficialis tendon rides superficial and splits at the proximal interphalangeal (PIP) joint, with a branch on either side of the profundus tendon, until its insertion on the middle phalanx. Throughout their course, starting at the metacarpophalangeal joint (MCP), several pulleys, numbered A1 to A5 from proximal to distal, secure both flexor tendons. These pulleys prevent bowstringing of the tendons with flexion. The dorsal aspect of the phalanges contains one extensor tendon: the extensor digitorum. This attaches to the middle phalanx but also contributes to the lateral band, which attaches laterally on the distal phalanx. The extensor hood, made up of transversely oriented sagittal bands at the MCP joint, stabilizes the extensor tendon.

The MCP and IP joints are synovial joints with synovial pouches proximal to the joint line on both the dorsal and volar aspects. The capsule is thicker on the volar aspect, where the volar plate reinforces it. The volar plate is made of thick fibrocartilage and limits finger hyperextension. The proper collateral and accessory collateral ligaments are two strong ligaments at both the ulnar and radial aspects of the joints. They reinforce and thicken the capsule on both sides of the joint. In the thumb, the ulnar collateral ligament (UCL) of the MCP joint is covered by the dorsal aponeurosis of the adductor pollicis muscle that inserts onto the dorsal aspect of the joint.

M.C. Bayes, M.D. (✉)
Crane Clinic for Sports Medicine, 219 Chesterfield Towne Plaza, Chesterfield, MO 63005, USA
e-mail: bayesmc32@hotmail.com

## Probe, Machine Settings, and Technique

A high-frequency transducer of at least 10 MHz is optimal for the hand and fingers owing to the superficial nature of the structures. A "hockey stick" probe, which has a small surface footprint, is also beneficial to maintain contact between the probe surface and the skin near the bony surfaces of the hand and fingers. Most ultrasound machines have preset musculoskeletal settings to improve superficial structure visualization. As one is getting started imaging, it is recommended to use these presets for evaluation of the hand and finger.

The optimal way to evaluate the hand and fingers is with the patient in a seated position. Typically, the dorsal aspect is evaluated first, with the hand placed on a small block or cylinder with the fingers hanging over its edge to aid in dynamic imaging during extension. Copious use of ultrasound gel is necessary to maintain skin contact. Alternatively, a standoff pad may be used. An evaluation of the hand and fingers may be focused on the pathologic region, but it is wise to master the complete evaluation to learn normal variants vs. pathologic findings. Comparison with the contralateral hand is also useful.

## Common Pathologic Conditions

### Extensor Tendon Tear, Extensor Avulsion Fracture/Mallet Finger

During evaluation of a tendon over the phalanges, long-axis planes are useful for demonstrating focal areas of tendon swelling and for evaluating tendon gliding with dynamic examination. Ultrasound is useful to identify full-thickness tendon tears and to locate the retraction of the tendon end. Partial tears are seen as focal hypoechoic (dark) areas within the tendon. Most extensor tendon injuries occur due to sudden flexion on an actively extending distal phalanx, often avulsing the tip of bone with the tendon. As a result, the

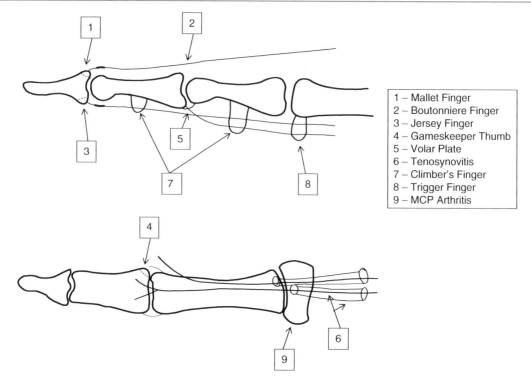

**Fig. 6.1** Common finger pathology

fingertip cannot be extended, causing a mallet finger deformity (Fig. 6.1 and Table 6.1).

## Central Slip Tear/Boutonniere Deformity

A boutonniere deformity occurs when the central slip of the extensor tendon tears at its insertion on the base of the middle phalanx. Longitudinal imaging shows the disruption in the tendon at the level of the PIP joint. The lateral slips of the extensor tendon move below the midline axis of the PIP joint to become PIP flexors. Because the lateral slips remain attached to the base of the distal phalanx, they lead to hyperextension of the distal IP joint (see Fig. 6.1 and Table 6.1).

## Flexor Tendon Tear/Jersey Finger

The flexor digitorum superficialis and/or the flexor digitorum profundus can tear. Avulsion of the flexor digitorum profundus from its distal insertion can occur as a result of a forced passive hyperextension injury on an actively flexed finger. This occurs usually during contact sports such as football or rugby and is commonly referred to as "jersey finger." This can cause an avulsion of a bony fragment from the palmar aspect of the distal phalanx, which commonly retracts (see Fig. 6.1 and Table 6.2).

## Volar Plate Injury

Volar plate injuries are typically due to hyperextension trauma of the joint. A long-axis view of the joint will show a hypoechoic cleft in the palmar plate if it is a full-thickness tear, just deep to the flexor tendon (see Fig. 6.1 and Table 6.2).

## Tenosynovitis

Tenosynovitis is characterized by distention of the synovial sheath around the tendon. If traumatic, a careful search for a hyperechoic structure within the tendon sheath should be performed because surgical removal is mandatory if a foreign body is found lying within a synovial sheath. Long-axis view of the sheath fluid is best done over the metacarpal head owing to the more superficial course of the flexor tendons. Short-axis view gives a clear assessment of the volume of tendon sheath fluid (see Fig. 6.1 and Table 6.2).

## Annular Pulley Tear/Climber's Finger

Acute tears of the annular pulleys are mainly due to maximal resisted flexion of the fingers, a common injury in rock climbers. The A2 and A4 pulleys are most commonly affected.

**Table 6.1** Hand and finger: dorsal view of finger

| Patient position | Transducer position and description | Picture of scan and labeled structures | Pearls/pitfalls |
| --- | --- | --- | --- |
| *Extensor tendon* Patient seated, hand resting with fingers extended, dorsal side up | 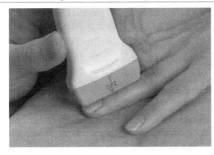 Long-axis view Probe over DIP, align with longitudinal extensor tendon fibers | 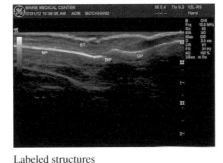 Labeled structures ET—extensor tendon and its insertion onto the DP—distal phalanx MP—middle phalanx DIP—distal interphalangeal joint | If avulsion is present, must identify and treat appropriately to avoid mallet finger deformity at the DIP joint. May place hand on a small cylinder with fingers over its edge to aid in dynamic testing of extension |
| *Extensor tendon central slip* Similar positioning as above | 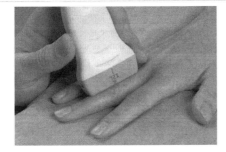 Long-axis view Similar to extensor tendon, probe is long axis over dorsal PIP/proximal aspect of middle phalanx | 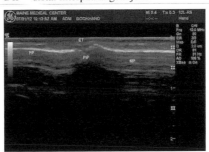 Labeled structures ET—extensor tendon PP—proximal phalanx MP—middle phalanx PIP—proximal interphalangeal joint | If full-thickness central slip tear, must manage correctly to avoid boutonniere deformity due to volar migration of the lateral bands of the extensor tendon |

**Table 6.2** Hand and finger: palmar or volar view of the finger

| Patient position | Transducer position and description | Picture of scan and labeled structures | Pearls/pitfalls |
| --- | --- | --- | --- |
| *Flexor digitorum profundus* Patient seated, with volar aspect of hand up | 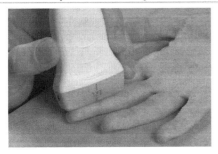 Long-axis view Probe is long axis centered over the flexor tendon and underlying volar plate at the PIP joint | 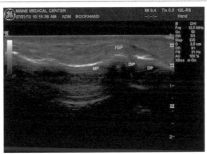 Labeled structures FDP—flexor digitorum profundus DP—distal phalanx MP—middle phalanx DIP—distal interphalangeal joint | Tendon visible as it inserts in the distal phalanx If full-thickness tear of the FDP, the patient is unable to actively flex the DIP joint against resistance Clinician must find the proximally migrated avulsion fragment/torn tendon; may migrate proximal into the hand. Surgical referral is necessary |

(continued)

**Table 6.2** (continued)

| Patient position | Transducer position and description | Picture of scan and labeled structures | Pearls/pitfalls |
|---|---|---|---|
| *Flexor digitorum superficialis* Patient seated, with volar aspect of hand up | 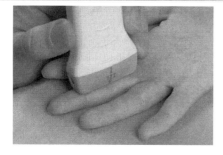 Long-axis view Probe is long axis centered over the flexor tendon, at the PIP joint | 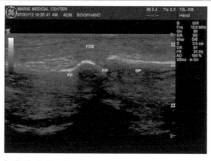 Labeled structures FDS—flexor digitorum superficialis PP—proximal phalanx MP—middle phalanx PIP—proximal interphalangeal joint | Tendon visible as it inserts in the middle phalanx If full-thickness tear of the FDS, the patient is unable to actively flex the PIP joint against resistance Clinician must find the proximally migrated avulsion fragment/torn tendon; may migrate proximal into the hand. Surgical referral is necessary |
| *Volar plate* Patient seated, with volar aspect of hand up | 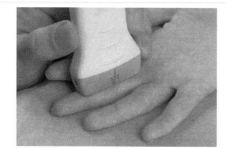 Long-axis view Probe is long axis centered over the volar plate of PIP joint | 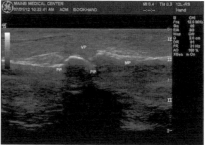 Labeled structures VP—volar plate PP—proximal phalanx MP—middle phalanx PIP—proximal interphalangeal joint | Volar plate is identified as structure spanning the two phalanx of the DIP joint |
| *Annular pulley* Patient seated, with volar aspect of hand up | 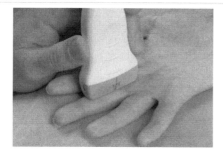 Long-axis view Probe is long axis over the proximal phalanx | 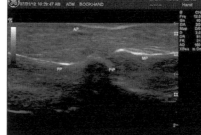 Labeled structures FT—flexor tendon AP—annular pulley PP—proximal phalanx MP—middle phalanx PIP—proximal interphalangeal joint | Annular pulley injury confirmed with active resisted flexion causing obvious separation of the flexor tendon from the proximal phalanx; confirmed with comparison of adjacent finger |
| *A1 pulley* Patient seated, with volar aspect of hand up | 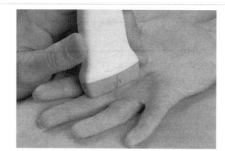 Long-axis view Probe is long axis over the MCP joint in the palm | 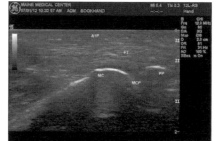 Labeled structures FT—flexor tendon MC—metacarpal PP—proximal phalanx MCP—metacarpal phalangeal joint A1P—A1 pulley | Hypoechoic thickening of the A1 pulley with mild inferior deviation of the flexor tendon is indicative of trigger finger. Dynamic evaluation may show tendon catching in the pulley |

**Table 6.3** Hand and finger: evaluation of the MCP joint

| Patient position | Transducer position and description | Picture of scan and labeled structures | Pearls/pitfalls |
|---|---|---|---|
| *MCP* Patient seated, with dorsal aspect of hand up | 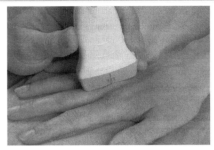 Long-axis view Probe is long axis over the MCP joint | 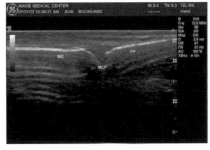 Labeled structures MCP—metacarpal phalangeal joint PP—proximal phalanx MC—metacarpal | Osteophytes, synovial distention, and effusion are all symptoms of arthritis |

A missed diagnosis can lead to a flexion contracture of the PIP joint and secondary osteoarthritis. The easiest way to diagnose this is by viewing a subluxing flexor tendon that instead of coursing along the concavity of the phalanges lies at a variable distance from the volar cortex. This is best done by scanning during active flexion while the examiner tries to extend it by gently pushing the fingertip (see Fig. 6.1 and Table 6.2).

## A1 Pulley Thickening/Trigger Finger

Chronic repetitive movement of the finger may lead to thickening of the A1 pulley and impingement of the involved tendon in the narrowed digital tunnel. A long-axis view at the level of the MCP joint shows hypoechoic thickening of the A1 pulley and mild deviation of the flexor tendon (see Fig. 6.1 and Table 6.2).

## MCP/IP Joint Arthritis

Ultrasound is highly sensitive in detecting joint effusion and small osteophytes and bony erosions that are often missed on standard radiographs. Effusion is visible as synovial distention with underlying hypoechoic fluid (see Fig. 6.1 and Table 6.3).

## Collateral Ligament Tear/Gamekeeper's Thumb

Assessment of the collateral ligaments of the second through fifth MCPs can be difficult. The most common and important collateral ligament injury is a tear of the UCL at the thumb MCP joint. An acute injury is referred to as a skier's thumb, while a chronic injury is referred to as a gamekeeper's thumb. The mechanism is excessive flexion and valgus stress, which leads to distal tear of the ligament (see Fig. 6.1 and Table 6.3).

US images should be obtained at rest and during cautious valgus stress to assess for increased radial subluxation of the proximal phalanx. Care should be taken to avoid causing displacement of a non-displaced ligament tear (Table 6.4).

With a first MCP UCL tear, care should be taken to differentiate a sesamoid bone from a cortical avulsion of the base of the proximal phalanx. Seeing the rounded appearance of the sesamoid bone easily does this. A long-axis image at the level of the metacarpal head is used to detect a displaced proximal ligament fragment (Stener lesion) over the proximal edge of the adductor pollicis aponeurosis. The torn end of the ligament "bunches" up and gives the appearance of a "yo-yo on a string." This lesion has surgical ramifications and is not to be missed (see Fig. 6.1 and Table 6.4).

## Red Flags

Failure to correctly diagnose an extensor tendon avulsion fracture can result in a permanent mallet finger deformity with loss of extension at the DIP joint. Missing an extensor tendon central slip tear at its insertion on the base of the middle phalanx can lead to a boutonniere deformity with a fixed hyperextended DIP joint and flexed PIP joint. A tear of the insertion of the flexor digitorum profundus that is missed can lead to worsening proximal retraction of the free end of the tendon from its insertion point, making repair more difficult or impossible. In the evaluation of a thumb MCP joint UCL injury, one must take care not to use excessive force during dynamic testing. If one is not careful, the dynamic test can inadvertently lead to ligament displacement, which means transforming a noncomplicated tear into a displaced lesion requiring surgery. Also, missing a displaced ligament rupture (Stener lesion) will lead to permanent instability and degenerative changes of the MCP joint. A missed annular pulley tear diagnosis, such as climber's finger, can lead to permanent flexion contracture of the IP joint and secondary arthritis.

**Table 6.4** Hand and finger: thumb

| Patient position | Transducer position and description | Picture of scan and labeled structures | Pearls/pitfalls |
|---|---|---|---|
| *UCL of thumb MCP joint* Patient seated, hand holding a rolled-up towel, thumb slightly abducted. Then examiner may apply gentle valgus stress | 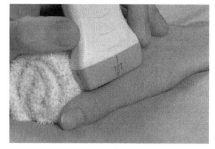 Probe is long axis over the MCP joint to provide a coronal view (long axis to UCL) | 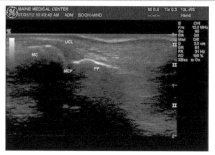 Normal UCL Labeled structures MC—metacarpal PP—proximal phalanx MCP—metacarpal phalangeal joint UCL—ulnar collateral ligament | When evaluating for possible UCL tear at the thumb MCP joint, the examiner must take care to first evaluate under ultrasound, if a full-thickness tear is easily visible. The examiner may apply gentle valgus stress to the MCP joint to assess for laxity and radial subluxation of the proximal phalanx on the metacarpal. However, be careful when stressing the joint to avoid displacing a proximally retracted UCL fragment under the adductor aponeurosis (Stener lesion) Comparison to the contralateral side is important when assessing joint laxity In long-axis view, full tear appears as gap in UCL, proximal retraction of UCL fragment appears balled up/ hyperechoic with overlying visible adductor aponeurosis |
|  | 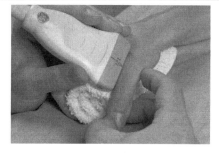 Long-axis view Stress view of UCL, probe same orientation | 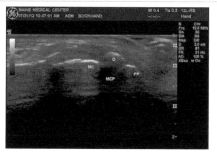 Chronic tear UCL, MCP opening with osteophyte Labeled structures MC—metacarpal PP—proximal phalanx MCP—metacarpal phalangeal joint O—osteophyte |  |

## Pearls and Pitfalls

Anisotropy must be avoided when evaluating for tendonosis or tendon tears. A hypoechoic appearing tendon may in fact be normal; the hypoechoic appearance may be due to the angle of the sound beam with relation to the structure being evaluated. This can be ruled out by moving the transducer so as to change this angle while evaluating the tendon for a more normal appearance. Positioning is key during the ultrasound examination. It is recommended to have both the patient and physician seated for the hand and finger evaluation, starting with the dorsal hand and moving in a systematic fashion. Having a small ball or cylinder to rest the fingers on is crucial. Correctly labeling and saving each image is very important.

## Suggested Reading

Bianchi S, Martinoli C. Ultrasound of the musculoskeletal system. New York: Springer; 2007.

Daniels JM, Zook EG, Lynch JM. Hand and wrist injuries: Part I. Nonemergent evaluation. Am Fam Physician. 2004a;69(8):1941–8.

Daniels JM, Zook EG, Lynch JM. Hand and wrist injuries: Part II. Emergent evaluation. Am Fam Physician. 2004b;69(8):1949–56.

Jacobson J. Fundamentals of musculoskeletal ultrasound. Philadelphia: Elsevier; 2007.

McNally E. Practical musculoskeletal ultrasound. Philadelphia: Elsevier; 2005.

# Wrist

Joseph J. Albano

## Approach to the Joint

### Volar Aspect of the Wrist

Have the patient seated with the hand on the table in a palm-up position. The examiner can be seated on an adjustable rolling stool. It is helpful if the table is also adjustable. For procedures, a small roll can be used to support the dorsal wrist to allow easier needle access. A rolled-up towel or chucks held together with tape would suffice.

Evaluate the proximal carpal tunnel first. Start with the transducer at the level of the wrist crease in a transverse (axial) position; this is short axis to the flexor tendons. Adjust the probe orientation so that one edge is over the scaphoid tubercle and the other is over the pisiform. Angle the transducer to compensate for the normal wrist contour. In addition, evaluate dynamic imaging with finger flexion and extension to demonstrate the normal motion of the tendons.

Now evaluate the distal carpal tunnel by moving the transducer distally until the trapezial tubercle (on the radial side) and the hook of the hamate (on the ulnar side) are visible. Slightly adjust probe orientation to account for changes in the median nerve depth. Slight wrist flexion can also maximize the image quality. Sweep the transducer from the proximal to distal carpal tunnel, systematically examining the median nerve from the distal radius to beyond the retinaculum. Note any increase in cross-sectional area (CSA) of the median nerve or anatomic variants, such as bifid median nerve or persistent median artery. Also examine the other structures noted above.

J.J. Albano, M.D. (✉)
Department of Regenerative Medicine, Comprehensive Orthopedics and Sports Medicine, 82 South 1100 East, Suite 303,
Salt Lake City, UT 84102, USA
e-mail: Skull466@gmail.com

Finally, evaluate Guyon's canal (ulnar artery, vein, and nerve) by moving the transducer medially (ulnar direction) using the pisiform bone as a landmark.

### Dorsal Aspect of the Wrist

The patient can remain seated and place the hand on the table, with the hand and wrist halfway between pronation and supination and the thumb toward the ceiling. Then place the probe on the radial styloid, transverse, or short axis, to the radius. The first dorsal compartment (abductor pollicis longus [APL] ventral and extensor pollicis longus [EPL] dorsal) can be scanned. The APL should be followed distally to the scaphoid to assess its accessory tendons. The radial artery and sensory branch of the radial nerve can also be evaluated in this position.

The patient then turns the wrist, so the palm is facing downward to view the second dorsal compartment. The extensor carpi radialis longus (ECRL) and the extensor carpi radialis brevis (ECRB) are evaluated by moving the probe, transverse (short-axis position), toward the radial styloid. The probe is then swept (slowly) proximally to view where the second compartment intersects with the first dorsal compartment. Tendinopathy here may indicate intersection syndrome.

The probe is then brought distally to the center of the wrist over Lister's tubercle (LT) and placed in a transverse (short-axis position), centered over LT. Just radial is the ECRB (second compartment) and just to the ulnar aspect of the LT is the EPL, in the third dorsal compartment.

The probe, still transverse, can continue to be moved in an ulnar direction, and adjacent to the EPL is the fourth dorsal compartment (extensor indicis proprius [EIP] and the extensor digitorum communis [EDC] tendons). The extensor digiti quarti, or fifth compartment, is located between the ulna and radius. When the probe is completely over the distal ulna, it may need to be placed, short axis, on the ulnar side of the wrist to view the last extensor compartment, the extensor carpi ulnaris (ECU), a tendon that is commonly injured.

J.M. Daniels and W.W. Dexter (eds.), *Basics of Musculoskeletal Ultrasound*,
DOI 10.1007/978-1-4614-3215-9_7, © Springer Science+Business Media New York 2013

The dorsal aspect of the wrist is fairly easy to scan, but at first the anatomy can be confusing. Memorization of the names of the tendons is not required at first. Each tendon can eventually be followed along its course, but to start, simply identify Lister's tubercle, and the six compartments can easily be scanned using Table 7.1 as a guide. As you become more comfortable, evaluation of ligaments and bones is possible in this area.

**Table 7.1** Wrist

| Patient position | Transducer position and description | Picture of scan and labeled structures | Pearls/pitfalls |
|---|---|---|---|
| **Volar wrist: proximal carpal tunnel** Patient is seated with the hand on the table with the palm up. It is helpful to place a small roll under the dorsal wrist for support. A small towel, rolled up and held together with tape, would suffice | 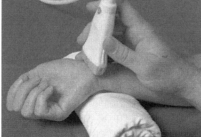 Proximal wrist crease, short axis Place the transducer over the proximal volar crease in a short-axis position. Adjust the probe orientation so that one edge is over the scaphoid tubercle on the radial side and the other is over the pisiform on the ulnar side. Scan the median nerve, FDS, FDP, FCR, palmaris longus, and scaphoid bone For all of these areas, scan in short- and long-axis planes | 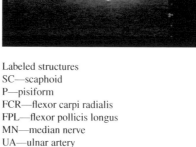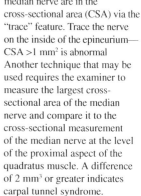 Labeled structures SC—scaphoid P—pisiform FCR—flexor carpi radialis FPL—flexor pollicis longus MN—median nerve UA—ulnar artery FDS—flexor digitorum profundus FDP—flexor digitorum profundus | Dynamic imaging with active finger flexion and extension demonstrates the normal motion of the tendons **Diagnosing carpal tunnel syndrome** Short-axis measurements of the median nerve are in the cross-sectional area (CSA) via the "trace" feature. Trace the nerve on the inside of the epineurium— CSA >1 mm$^2$ is abnormal Another technique that may be used requires the examiner to measure the largest cross-sectional area of the median nerve and compare it to the cross-sectional measurement of the median nerve at the level of the proximal aspect of the quadratus muscle. A difference of 2 mm$^3$ or greater indicates carpal tunnel syndrome. |
| | 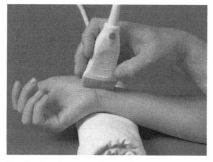 Proximal wrist crease, long axis | 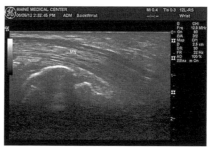 Labeled structures MN—median nerve | **Longitudinal median nerve** Compression neuropathy may appear as a dumbbell or peanut with a larger nerve distally and proximally. A smaller nerve is at the compressed site. Dynamically assess the tendons with flexion and extension |
| **Volar wrist: distal carpal tunnel** Patient is seated with the hand on the table with the palm up. It is helpful to place a small roll under the dorsal wrist for support. A small towel or chucks, rolled up and held together with tape, would suffice | 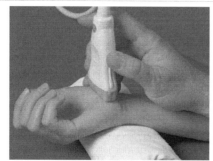 Wrist crease, short axis Move the transducer distally until the trapezial tubercle is on the radial side and the hook of the hamate is on the ulnar side. Sweep the transducer from the proximal to distal carpal tunnel, systematically examining the median nerve and the tendons from the distal radius to beyond the retinaculum. Note any increase in cross-sectional area of the median nerve or anatomic variants, such as bifid median nerve or persistent median artery | 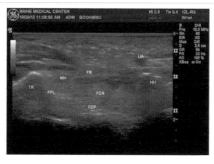 Labeled structures TR—trapezium HH—hook of hamate FPL—flexor pollicis longus MN—median nerve UA—ulnar artery FDS—flexor digitorum profundus FDP—flexor digitorum profundus FR—flexor retinaculum | Slightly adjust probe orientation to account for changes in the median nerve depth. Slight wrist flexion can also maximize the image quality Don't mistake the palmaris longus tendon, which lies superficial to the retinaculum, with the median nerve, which is deep to the retinaculum. In some people, the palmaris longus may not exist The radial artery and veins lie just radial to the flexor carpi radialis tendon. Ganglion cysts will be seen in this area as the transducer is moved proximal to distal In the long-axis view, the characteristic peanut-shaped or bilobed bony contours of the scaphoid bone are identified deep to the flexor carpi radialis (FCR) tendon. Fractures may be identified as cortical step-offs |

(continued)

**Table 7.1** (continued)

| Patient position | Transducer position and description | Picture of scan and labeled structures | Pearls/pitfalls |
|---|---|---|---|
| **Volar wrist: Guyon's canal** Patient is seated with the hand on the table with the palm up. It is helpful to place a small roll under the dorsal wrist for support. A small towel rolled up and held together with tape would suffice | 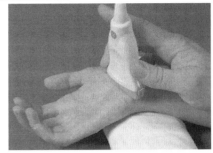 Distal wrist crease, ulnar aspect, short axis Move the transducer toward the ulna using the pisiform bone as a landmark | 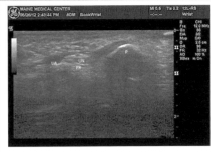 Labeled structures P—pisiform UA—ulnar artery UN—ulnar nerve FR—flexor retinaculum | The ulnar artery is on the radial side, and the ulnar nerve is on the ulnar side of the tunnel next to the pisiform. There are two branches of the ulnar nerve: the superficial sensory branch and the deep motor branch. The latter lies over the hook of the hamate |
| **Dorsal wrist: 1st compartment** The hand is placed halfway between pronation and supination, with the radius superior and 90° to the table | 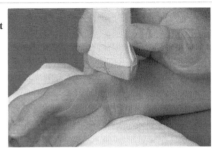 Short-axis view | 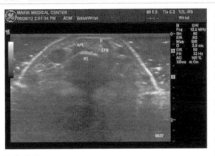 Labeled structures R—retinaculum RS—radial styloid APL—abductor pollicis longus EPB—extensor pollicis brevis | Abductor pollicis longus (APL) (volar) and extensor pollicis brevis (EPB) (dorsal) tendons over the radial styloid. The radial nerve and artery lie outside the compartment and move from ventral to dorsal over these tendons To remember the tendons in the first, second, and third compartments, moving from radial to ulna, think alternating thoughts: longus-brevis-longus-brevis-longus (APL, EPB, ECRL [extensor carpi radialis longus], ECRB [extensor carpi radialis brevis], EPL [extensor pollicis longus]). It also goes from abductor to extensor and pollicis to carpi and back to pollicis |
| | 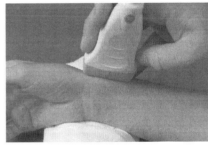 Long-axis view | 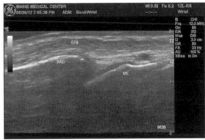 Labeled structures RAD—radius MC—metacarpal EPB—extensor pollicis brevis | |
| **Dorsal wrist: 2nd compartment** Patient is seated with the hand on the table with the palm up. It is helpful to place a small roll under the dorsal wrist for support. A small towel, rolled up and held together with tape, would suffice | 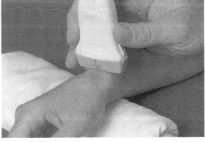 Short-axis view Position the transducer slightly toward the ulna | 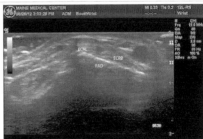 Labeled structures RAD—radius ECRL—extensor carpi radialis longus ECRB—extensor carpi radialis brevis | **Intersection syndrome** Clinical symptoms or US findings where the APL and EPB of the first compartment cross over at the "intersection" of the ECRL and ECRB |

**Table 7.1** (continued)

| Patient position | Transducer position and description | Picture of scan and labeled structures | Pearls/pitfalls |
|---|---|---|---|
| | 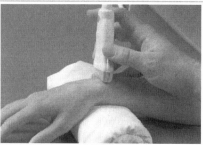<br>Short-axis view<br>Move cranially over the ECRL and ECRB tendons until the APL and EPB of the first compartment cross over at the "intersection" | 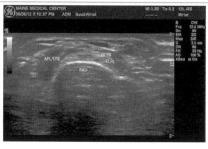<br>Labeled structures<br>As above, and APL/EPB—abductor pollicis longus and extensor pollicis brevis | |
| **Dorsal wrist:**<br>**3rd compartment**<br>The hand is placed palm down for the 3rd to 5th compartments | 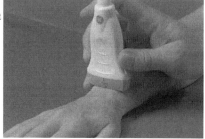<br>Short-axis view<br>The transducer is placed over the middorsal wrist for evaluation of these compartments | 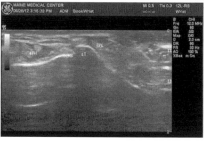<br>Labeled structures<br>LT—Lister's tubercle<br>EPL—extensor pollicis longus<br>ECRB—extensor carpi radialis brevis<br>4TH—fourth compartment | Lister's tubercle over the dorsal radius separates the second compartment (which is radial) from the third compartment (which is ulnar)<br>Follow the extensor pollicis longus tendon from the ulnar side of Lister's tubercle as it crosses the ECRB and ECRL tendons down to the insertion on the distal phalanx of the thumb |
| **Dorsal wrist:**<br>**4th and 5th compartments**<br>The hand is placed palm down for the 4th to 5th compartments | As above. Transducer is moved incrementally toward ulna | 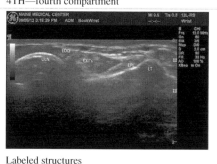<br>Labeled structures<br>LT—Lister's tubercle<br>ULN—ulna<br>EXTs—extensor tendons (extensor digitorum communis, extensor indicis proprius)<br>EPL—extensor pollicis longus<br>EDQ—extensor digiti quinti | |
| **Dorsal wrist:**<br>**scapholunate ligament**<br>Palm down with ulnar deviation to assess the ligament integrity | Short-axis view<br>From the level of Lister's tubercle on the radius, sweep the transducer distal until the scaphoid comes into view. Then move the probe ulnarly until the lunate is also brought into view. Between these bones is the triangular SL ligament<br>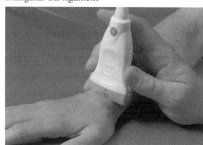 | 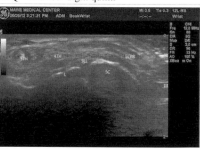<br>Labeled structures<br>L—lunate<br>SC—scaphoid<br>ECRB—extensor carpi radialis brevis<br>SLL—scapholunate ligament<br>4TH, 5TH—fourth and fifth compartments with extensor tendons | **Scapholunate ligament**<br>The SL ligament may be visualized from both the dorsal and volar directions. However, the dorsal aspect is easily visualized. SL tears may be seen in this view as hypoechoic areas in the hyperechoic ligament<br>Dorsal wrist ganglion cysts typically appear superficial to the SL ligament |

(continued)

**Table 7.1** (continued)

| Patient position | Transducer position and description | Picture of scan and labeled structures | Pearls/pitfalls |
|---|---|---|---|
| **Dorsal wrist: longitudinal** Palm down | The transducer is placed long axis to the extensor tendons. Note: Scan from the radial to the ulnar aspect of wrist to assess entire dorsum 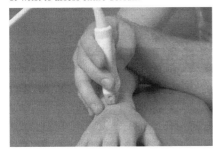 | 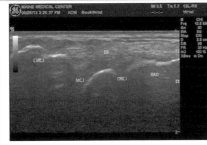 Labeled structures ER—extensor retinaculum RAD—radius CMCJ—carpometacarpal joint DRCJ—distal radiocarpal joint MCJ—midcarpal joint | The extensor retinaculum has an oblique course, proximally from the radius distally past the ulna. It is hyperechoic and can measure up to 1.7 mm thick by 23 mm wide. It may appear hypoechoic due to anisotropy if the oblique course is not considered The dorsal radiocarpal, midcarpal, and carpometacarpal (CMC) joint recesses are evaluated for effusion, synovial hypertrophy, osteophytes, and bony erosion. Common locations for osteoarthritis are the first CMC and radiocarpal joints |
| **Dorsal wrist: sixth compartment** The hand is placed in extreme pronation with the thumb on the table | The transducer is placed over the ulnar styloid, first in an axial plane (short axis to the ulna) then in a longitudinal plane (long axis to ulna) and then moved distally 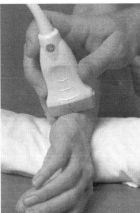 Short-axis view 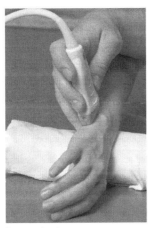 Long-axis view | 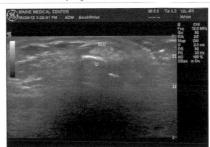 Labeled structures U—ulna ECU—extensor carpi ulnaris 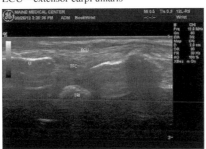 Labeled structures U—ulna TFC—triangular fibrocartilage ECU—extensor carpi ulnaris TRI—triquetrum | The triangular fibrocartilage complex (TFCC) consists of the triangular fibrocartilage, the meniscal homologue, the ECU tendon sheath, and the volar and dorsal radiocarpal ligaments. Look at the TFCC for hypo- to anechoic areas that may signify a tear |

(continued)

**Table 7.1** (continued)

| Patient position | Transducer position and description | Picture of scan and labeled structures | Pearls/pitfalls |
|---|---|---|---|
| **Dorsal wrist: distal radioulnar joint (DRUJ)** Palm down | The transducer is placed short axis to the DRUJ and more proximal than the joint line | 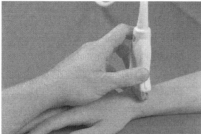 Labeled structures DRUJ—distal radial ulnar joint U—ulna R—radius 4TH, 5TH—4th and 5th compartments with extensor tendons | |

## Probe Selection and Presets

Because the structures are superficial, a high-frequency linear transducer of 10–13 MHz is required. Thick transducer gel or standoff pad should be used to aid in this process. A "hockey stick" transducer can be helpful for the smaller structures. If your machine has wrist or hand presets, start with those.

## Common Problems

### I Can't Find the Median Nerve!

When imaged in the short-axis, or transverse, plane, normal peripheral nerves have a characteristic honeycomb appearance. The fascicles are hypoechoic, and the surrounding connective tissue is hyperechoic. If it is difficult to identify the median nerve, move the transducer proximally. Knowledge of the characteristic location, course, echogenicity, and anisotropy will assist in the identification.

The median nerve lies superficial to the flexor digitorum profundus and superficialis tendons and deep to the flexor retinaculum. The distal end of the nerve is tapered. Do not confuse the palmaris longus tendon with the median nerve. This tendon lies superficial to the retinaculum. The median nerve moves medial to lateral as it progresses distally from the proximal wrist crease.

The median nerve appears relatively hyperechoic proximally and hypoechoic distally. This is secondary to the relative echogenicity of the surrounding tissue. The muscle is hypoechoic proximally, and the tendons are hyperechoic distally. In order to take advantage of the change in echogenicity of the tendons, angle the transducer to produce a hypoechoic signal in the normally hyperechoic tendons. The median nerve should remain hypoechoic.

## How Do I Diagnose Carpal Tunnel Syndrome?

Carpal tunnel syndrome (CTS) findings on US include enlarged median nerve, bulging of the transverse carpal ligament, flattening ratio of the median nerve in the distal carpal tunnel and median nerve hypoechogenicity, and decreased mobility. The most commonly used criteria for diagnosing CTS with US imaging is the median nerve CSA. There is a lack of consensus in the literature regarding the most appropriate median nerve threshold to establish this diagnosis while scanning. Keep the transducer pressure minimal during measurements in order to avoid any pressure on the nerve. Some US machines have an ellipse tool, which uses a formula to create the CSA. This *indirect method* is not the chosen method for median nerve CSA measurement. *Direct tracing* of the nerve inside the epineurium is more accurate. Using this method, Ziswiler et al. [1] derived a cutoff value of 10 mm$^2$ and achieved a sensitivity of 82 % and specificity of 87 %, which approaches those of electrodiagnostic tests. For a median nerve CSA <8 mm$^2$, CTS can be ruled out. For CSA >12 mm$^2$, CTS can be ruled in. Klauser et al. [2] described a more accurate method. In this method, the carpal tunnel was scanned from the proximal portion (scaphoid-pisiform level) to the distal portion (trapezium-hamate level). The largest median nerve cross-sectional area (CSAc) measurement was used. The more proximal cross-sectional area (CSAp) measurement was obtained in the distal forearm at the level of the proximal third of the pronator quadratus muscle. The median nerve lies between the flexor pollicis longus and flexor digitorum superficialis tendons in this location. The value for the difference between CSAc and CSAp is delta CSA. The best diagnostic discrimination was achieved using a delta CSA threshold of 2 mm², which yielded 99 % sensitivity and 100 % specificity. The appearance of a compressed median nerve may be similar to a dumbbell or peanut with the larger swollen nerve proximally and distally and a smaller compressed nerve in the middle (see Table 7.1).

## What Are the Findings of De Quervain's Tenosynovitis?

The APL and extensor pollicis brevis (EPB) tendons lie in the first dorsal compartment. The sheath or tendons may become irritated with repetitive motion and overuse. The classic findings of tenosynovitis should be seen, which include an anechoic (black) area surrounding the tendon and hyperemia (increased vascularity upon Doppler imaging). Tendinosis (thickened and hypoechoic [darker] tendon) or even an intrasubstance tear may be seen in these tendons.

## What Is Intersection Syndrome?

The APL and EPB of the first compartment cross over the ECRL and ECRB of the second compartment approximately 4 cm proximal to the Lister's tubercle. Symptoms may occur at this intersection due to overuse and the associated friction of these tendons.

## Red Flags

Don't ever put a needle into an anechoic space that turns out to be an artery or an aneurysm. Always check for flow using power Doppler imaging or color flow.

## Pearls and Pitfalls

- When first learning this wrist exam, it is helpful to practice a complete exam of all of the areas, volar and dorsal. However, during a time-crunched day at the office, it is acceptable to focus the US exam over the clinically relevant area. You will not miss a diagnosis focusing your exam in this way.
- Volar. Don't miss a scaphoid fracture! With the transducer in the longitudinal plane over the flexor carpi radialis tendon, the characteristic peanut-shaped or bilobed bony contours of the scaphoid bone are identified deep to the tendon. Fractures appear as cortical step-offs.
- Dorsal scapholunate (SL) ligament tear. The SL ligament may be visualized from both the dorsal and volar directions. However, the dorsal aspect is more easily visualized. SL tears may be seen in this view as hypoechoic areas in the hyperechoic ligament.
- Look for dorsal wrist ganglion cysts superficial to the SL ligament.
- The triangular fibrocartilage complex (TFCC) consists of the triangular fibrocartilage, the meniscal homologue, the ECU tendon sheath, and the volar and dorsal radiocarpal ligaments. Look at the TFCC for hypo- to anechoic areas, which signify a tear.

## Clinical Exercise

1. Place the probe on the palmar side of the wrist. Identify the median nerve at the CSA between the scaphoid and pisiform and the trapezium and hook of hamate. Trace the outline of the nerve with your measurement setting and record. Now place the probe more proximally along the forearm to the pronator quadratus muscle. Take a cross-sectional measurement of the median nerve there and record it.
2. Place the transducer on Lister's tubercle in a transverse (short-axis) plane. Begin moving the transducer ulnarward and radial-ward. Identify as many cross-sections of the six extensor tendon compartments as possible. There are two (first and second) compartments radial to Lister's tubercle and the other four are ulnar.

## References

1. Ziswiler HR, Reichenbach S, Vögelin E, Bachmann LM, Villiger PM, Jüni P. Diagnostic value of sonography in patients with suspected carpal tunnel syndrome: a prospective study. Arthritis Rheum. 2005;52(1):304–11.
2. Klauser AS, Halpern EJ, De Zordo T, Feuchtner GM, Arora R, Gruber J, et al. Carpal tunnel syndrome assessment with US: value of additional cross-sectional area measurements of the median nerve in patients versus healthy volunteers. Radiology. 2009;250(1):171–7.

# Elbow

8

### Pierre d'Hemecourt

## Approach to the Joint

The elbow is divided into four regions arbitrarily for convenience. In a limited exam, not all of the areas need to be imaged. These are the anterior, medial, lateral, and posterior regions. Examination of these areas are most easily done in the seated position but may be performed in the supine (laying down, face up) position. When interventional procedures are done, they are best done in the supine position. When the patient is seated, the involved arm is next to the stretcher or examining table. Both patient and clinician are optimally on stools with rollers, with the clinician stool slightly more elevated. This allows the clinician to make slight adjustments to positions of both chairs. The clinician is facing the patient with the ultrasound unit on the opposite side of the imaged elbow. When the patient is supine, the clinician is on the side of the affected elbow with the ultrasound unit on the opposite side of the bed facing the clinician. The elbow may be placed on a small pillow or folded towel.

The anterior elbow is viewed with the elbow extended or slightly flexed. In this position, dynamic imaging of the anterior recess with flexion and extension may be performed, looking for excess intra-articular fluid. Pronation and supination may be used to visualize the distal biceps region.

The medial elbow is visualized with an abducted and externally rotated forearm (supination). Elbow flexion is variable by patient comfort but is usually about 30°.

The lateral elbow is imaged with the arm adducted and internally rotated (fully pronated, palm down). Elbow flexion is between 20° and 40° on the table. This may also be accomplished by having both hands together with thumbs up and elbows fully extended.

The posterior elbow is visualized in several positions. Seated, the shoulder is flexed forward just above 90° with a fully flexed elbow. The cubical tunnel may be visualized. Alternately, the patient may extend the arm behind him with the elbow flexed at 90° and the palm down on the table. The patient's chair is elevated to make this more comfortable, and the examiner is standing behind the patient. This allows full view of the cubical tunnel and surrounding muscles. The cubital tunnel may also be viewed in the described medial approach.

## Anterior Elbow

The anterior elbow includes structures from the pronator teres attachment on the medial epicondyle to the brachioradialis. From medial to lateral, the more superficial structures include the median nerve, brachial artery, brachialis muscle, biceps brachii muscle and tendon, and radial nerve (Fig. 8.1). These are best visualized with an axial view of the elbow (transverse or short axis to long bones) scanning 5 cm above and below the joint. The brachial artery is easily visualized just lateral to the biceps brachii and noted with the pulsation and noncompressible nature (brachial vein is compressible). Just *medial* to the artery is the "honeycombed"-appearing median nerve. Just *lateral* to the artery is the median nerve, which is also "honeycombed" in appearance. Just medial to the artery is the brachialis muscle, which can be followed to its insertion on the coronoid process. The biceps tendon can also be followed to its insertion onto the radial tuberosity. Visualization of the bicep insertion is an important clinical point discussed later. Lateral to the biceps muscle, the radial

P. d'Hemecourt, M.D. (✉)
Division of Sports Medicine, Primary Care Sports Medicine, Boston Children's Hospital, 319 Longwood Avenue, Boston, MA 02115, USA
e-mail: sports.medicine@childrens.harvard.edu;
Pierre.Dhemecourt@childrens.harvard.edu

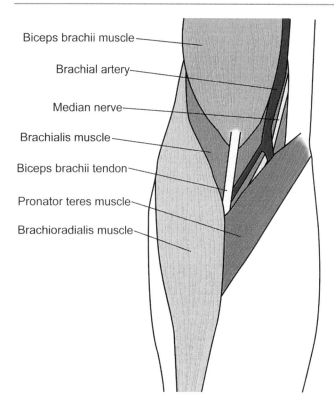

Biceps brachii muscle

Brachial artery

Median nerve

Brachialis muscle

Biceps brachii tendon

Pronator teres muscle

Brachioradialis muscle

**Fig. 8.1** Anterior structures of the elbow

Deep to the common flexor tendon is the anterior band of the UCL. This is the major restraint to valgus stress. It arises from the anterior aspect of the epicondyle and inserts medial to the coronoid process on the sublime tubercle. This band is the only reliable band of the UCL that is well visualized by ultrasound.

When imaging the medial structures, the longitudinal (long-axis) view over the epicondyle with the elbow in extension will demonstrate the UCL relatively hypoechoic to the common flexor tendon above (see Table 8.1). But if the elbow is in 90° of flexion with the abducted and externally rotated arm, the UCL will appear more hyperechoic.

## Lateral Elbow

Lateral elbow structures include the brachioradialis, extensor carpi radialis longus, the common extensor tendon, and the supinator muscles. The brachioradialis and extensor carpi radialis longus originate from the supracondylar ridge above the epicondyle separate from the common extensor tendon that inserts on the anterolateral aspect of the lateral epicondyle (Fig. 8.4). The deepest of the lateral group is the superficial and deep portions of the supinator muscles. The superficial muscle originates from the posterior aspect of the epicondyle, annular ligament, and ulna fossa. The deep head originates from the supinator fossa of the ulna. Together, they wrap around the radial neck and insert on the proximal radial shaft to assist the biceps in supination. The superficial portion in some individuals forms a fibrous band called the "arcade of Frohse." The PIN enters under the superficial head or, when present, the arcade of Frohse.

The common extensor tendon is comprised of the extensor carpi radialis brevis (comprising most of the deep tendon), the extensor digitorum communis (comprising most of the superficial tendon), extensor digiti minimi, and extensor carpi ulnaris. These are best viewed in a longitudinal view (long axis) anterolaterally over the radial head (see Table 8.1). The underlying lateral collateral ligament is difficult to differentiate from the common extensor tendon.

## Posterior Elbow

The posterior elbow is comprised of the cubital tunnel medially, the triceps muscle, and the anconeus muscle laterally, which originates on the lateral olecranon and inserts on the posterior aspect of the lateral epicondyle. The triceps tendon represents the convergence of the medial, lateral, and long head of the triceps. This inserts distal to the tip of the olecranon. The olecranon bursa lies dorsal to the olecranon.

nerve is found between the brachialis and brachioradialis. The nerve can be followed distally to where it divides into the more medial superficial branch and the deep posterior interosseous nerve (PIN), which traverses the supinator muscles at the radial neck (Table 8.1).

The deeper structures of the anterior elbow include the anterior recess, which appears as a concavity in the distal humerus and is comprised of the radial fossa (Fig. 8.2) and coronoid fossa. A fat pad normally resides in the fossa and may have a small amount of fluid behind the fat pad.

## Medial Elbow

The medial elbow includes the tendons of the medial epicondyle and the ulnar collateral ligament (UCL). The defining muscle is the pronator teres, which has two origins: one just proximal to the epicondyle and one on the ulnar aspect of the coronoid process. The median nerve traverses between these two origins of the pronator teres. Just medial to the pronator teres is the common flexor tendon inserting onto the medial epicondyle. This is comprised from lateral to medial of the flexor carpi radialis, palmaris longus, flexor digitorum superficialis, and flexor carpi ulnaris (Fig. 8.3).

**Table 8.1** Elbow

| Patient position | Transducer position and description | Image description and labeled structures | Pearls/pitfalls |
|---|---|---|---|
| Anterior elbow Patient seated with elbow extended on table. May use pillow for support | 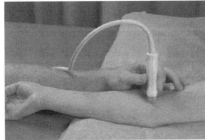 Transverse (or short-axis) view Scan from 5 cm above elbow to 5 cm below elbow | 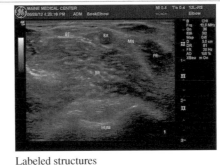 Labeled structures BT—biceps tendon BR—brachialis muscle BA—brachial artery MN—median nerve HUM—humerus/trochlea PR—pronator muscle | The radial nerve will split into the superficial branch medially and deeper branch laterally into the supinator muscle Supination and pronation will demonstrate the annular ligaments of the radial head as well as insertion of the biceps tendon |
| Anterior elbow | 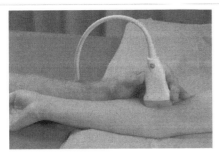 Longitudinal (or long-axis) view Scan across anterior elbow radial to ulnar aspect Radial sagittal | 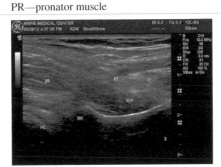 Labeled structures RH—radial head HC—humeral capitellum SUP—supinator BR—brachialis BT—biceps tendon | A small amount of fluid may be seen behind the fat pad of the radial and coronoid fossa and increased with elbow flexion The biceps tendon will demonstrate anisotropy artifact if the distal probe is not compressed as the tendon is followed more distally |
| Anterior elbow | 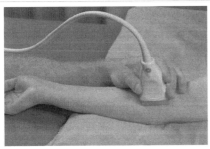 Long-axis view Ulna sagittal | 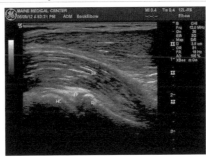 Labeled structures FP—fat pad BR—brachialis HC—humeral capitellum RH—radial head | Again, the fossa will demonstrate a small amount of fluid behind the fat pad Loose bodies can sometimes be identified with flexion and a small probe such as a "hockey-stick" probe The brachialis has a short tendon compared to the biceps |
| Medial elbow The seated patient holds the arm abducted and supinated with 20° elbow flexion. May use pillow for support | 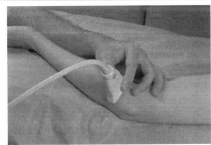 Short-axis view | 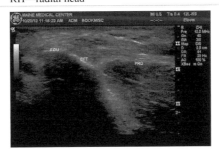 Labeled structures PRO—pronator teres CFT—common flexor tendon FCU—flexor carpi ulnaris | The pronator teres has two insertions: one above the epicondyle and one at the coronoid tuberosity |

(continued)

**Table 8.1** (continued)

| Patient position | Transducer position and description | Image description and labeled structures | Pearls/pitfalls |
|---|---|---|---|
| Medial elbow | 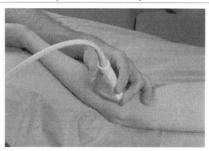<br>Long-axis view | 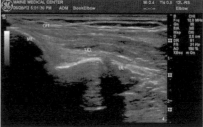<br>Labeled structures<br>ME—medial epicondyle<br>UCL—ulnar collateral ligament<br>CFT—common flexor tendon<br>UL—ulna | With 20° of flexion and valgus force, insufficiency of the UCL may be demonstrated but can be seen in asymptomatic throwers |
| Lateral elbow<br>The patient is seated with elbow flexed, pronated, and adducted. May use pillow for support | 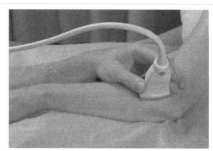<br>Long-axis view | 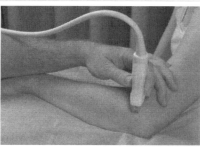<br>Labeled structures<br>LE—lateral epicondyle<br>RH—radial head<br>CET—common extensor tendon | |
| Lateral elbow | 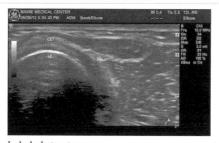<br>Short-axis view | 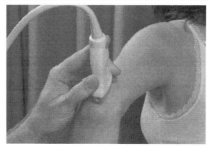<br>Labeled structures<br>CET—common extensor tendon<br>RN—radial nerve<br>LE—lateral epicondyle | The radial nerve is seen on the anterior and lateral views. On the lateral view, the deep branch at the supinator muscles is viewed for any impingement. This is first identified on short axis, and the probe then turns long axis over the nerve, looking for a sudden decrease in diameter. The radial nerve is identified at the arcade of Frohse |
| Posterior elbow<br>The patient is seated with the palm on the table and elbow flexion to 90° | 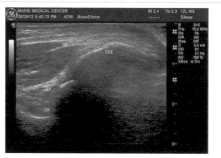<br>Long-axis view | Labeled structures<br>TT—triceps tendon<br>OLE—olecranon<br>FP—fat pad<br>OR—olecranon recess | Olecranon bursa is not noted unless it is inflamed |

(continued)

**Table 8.1** (continued)

| Patient position | Transducer position and description | Image description and labeled structures | Pearls/pitfalls |
|---|---|---|---|
| Posterior elbow | 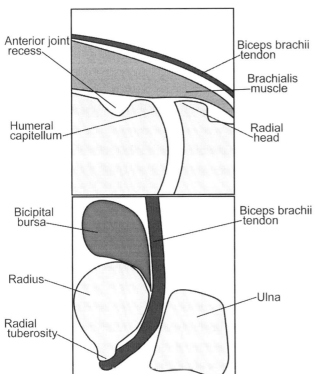Short-axis view | Labeled structures<br>UN—ulnar nerve<br>ME—medial epicondyle<br>OLE—olecranon<br>FCU—flexor carpi ulnaris<br>TT—triceps tendon | The cubital tunnel can be seen from a medial or posterior view. Dynamic flexion of the cubital tunnel is best done when seated with the medial view |

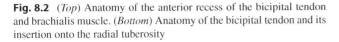

**Fig. 8.2** (*Top*) Anatomy of the anterior recess of the bicipital tendon and brachialis muscle. (*Bottom*) Anatomy of the bicipital tendon and its insertion onto the radial tuberosity

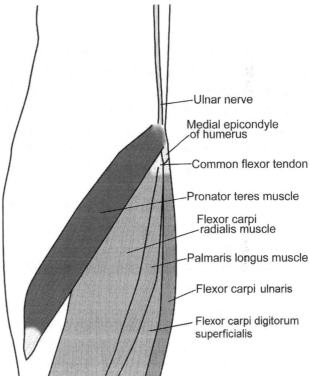

**Fig. 8.3** Medial structures of the elbow

The triceps tendon and olecranon bursa may be visualized in a longitudinal (long-axis) view.

Proximal to the cubital tunnel, the ulnar nerve enters a fibro-osseous groove (cubital groove) between the olecranon and epicondyle. The roof is a fibrous covering called Osborn's retinaculum or fascia and a floor formed by the posterior band of the UCL. In this space it is fairly mobile with flexion and extension. Distally, by about 1 cm, the nerve enters the true cubital tunnel between the two heads of the flexor carpi ulnaris, one from the olecranon and one from the medial epicondyle and one from the medial olecranon. The fibrous band between these two heads is an extension of Osborn's fascia ligament proximally, and it is referred to as the arcuate ligament (Fig. 8.5).

The ulnar nerve is best visualized in this groove with an axial view (transverse or short axis to nerve) and a small probe such as the hockey-stick probe (see Table 8.1). This allows for a dynamic exam of the ulnar nerve. As the elbow is slowly taken into full flexion, the medial triceps may cause subluxation of the nerve out of the groove.

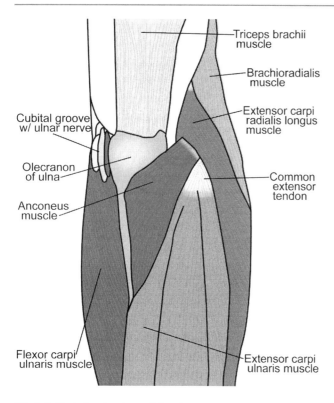

**Fig. 8.4** Posterior structures of the elbow

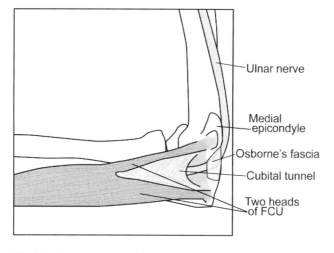

**Fig. 8.5** Deep structures of the elbow demonstrating the route of the ulnar nerve and sites of possible entrapment

## Probe Selection

A high-frequency probe is best for superficial structures like the elbow. A 5–15-MHz linear array transducer is used. A hockey-stick probe (5–10 MHz) may be useful around the medial and lateral elbow, especially for interventional procedures. This smaller probe will also allow easier dynamic flexion of the elbow.

## Specific Presets

A narrow field of view is best for these superficial structures. The focal zone should be set in a shallow range. The higher frequency range of the probe is usually set for most elbow structures. However, for the deeper structures, such as the distal biceps, or when looking in the recess for loose bodies, a lower setting is used for better visualization. Tissue harmonic imaging (THI) is a technique whereby the inherent tissue resonance is recorded. It may help differentiate different tissue layers such as the tendons inserting on the epicondyle. Finally, power Doppler imaging may be used to look for inflammation as well as neovascularization in tendinopathy.

## Common Problems

### Anterior Elbow

#### Distal Biceps

Common anterior elbow problems often involve the distal biceps, which includes biceps tendinopathy, rupture, or bicipitoradial bursitis (uncommon). The ultrasound probe should follow the tendon in a long-axis view to its insertion on the radial tuberosity with the elbow in full supination. This is a sagittal oblique plane. The probe should be kept parallel to the visualized tendon to avoid anisotropy artifact. This requires that the distal end of the probe be pushed gently into the soft tissue as the tendon turns deeper at the insertion. This will maintain a parallel configuration of the probe to the distal tendon. The probe may then be turned to an axial (transverse or short-axis) view of the tendon insertion, and possible bursa enlargement may be seen when the forearm is pronated. Ultrasound is unique compared to other imaging methods in this location because dynamic pronation and supination will demonstrate the bursa size change. The insertion site may also be viewed from a dorsal approach with the forearm pronated (see Table 8.1).

#### Posterior Interosseous Nerve Impingement

The deep branch of the radial nerve may be impinged at the edge of the superficial supinator muscle (arcade of Frohse), between the supinator muscles, by scar tissue or by a recurrent radial artery. This will often mimic lateral epicondylitis. It is best identified on an axial (transverse or short-axis) view above the elbow crease between the brachioradialis and brachialis (see Table 8.1). The axial (transverse or short-axis) view is followed down to the supinator muscles at the radial neck. The probe may then be turned to a longitudinal (long-axis) view of the nerve by centering the nerve and then slowly turning the probe, maintaining the nerve as the central focus. An impinged nerve will often appear swollen and hypoechoic above the area of constriction.

## Anterior Recess Assessment

Longitudinal (long-axis) views of the anterior recess are helpful in assessing the amount of joint effusion. Normally, a small amount of fluid may exist under the hyperechoic fat pad. Pathologic increases in effusion may be demonstrated by passively flexing the elbow. The smaller hockey-stick probe may be useful in this setting. Small loose bodies sometimes are visible with this technique of flexion and compression of the joint posteriorly. Chip fractures off the coronoid process may also be seen.

## Medial Elbow

### Medial Epicondylosis

The common flexor tendon may be predisposed to tendon degeneration with repetitive elbow valgus force combined with eccentric stresses of pronation and flexion from sports such as pitching and golf. This may present with medial elbow pain that is aggravated by resisted flexion and pronation. The ultrasound imaging may demonstrate partial tears or hypoechoic intrasubstance changes of the common flexor tendon. Insertional enthesopathy may demonstrate bony irregularities of the epicondyle. The power Doppler is useful to demonstrate neovascularization consistent with tendinopathy.

### Ulnar Collateral Ligament Injury

Injury to the UCL may occur with an acute injury such as an elbow dislocation. More commonly, it is secondary to an overuse valgus stress, such as with a baseball pitcher. It may present quite similarly to medial epicondylosis and may have coexisting tendinosis of the common flexor tendon. The UCL may be fully or partially torn. When partially torn, the ligament will demonstrate of thickening and hypoechoic changes. There can sometimes be some associated ligament calcification.

When the ligament is fully torn, a frank breach in the ligament may appear. Alternately, it may be manifested by soft-tissue indentation of the ligament. Widening of the joint or gapping of the UCL may be demonstrated with valgus stress.

## Lateral Elbow

### Lateral Epicondylosis

The common extensor tendon may be injured due to partial- or full-thickness tears. More commonly, it is involved in tendinosis with tendon degeneration and intrasubstance tearing. This is classically known as "tennis elbow" due the eccentric overload of the backhand. However, it is more commonly seen as a tendinosis of the nonathletic population and presents with lateral elbow pain worsened with wrist extension. Ultrasound imaging of the common extensor tendon most commonly demonstrates hypoechoic changes in the tendon distal to the insertion. The deeper extensor carpi radialis

brevis tendon is the most common area involved. However, insertional enthesopathy may also be demonstrated with bony irregularities on the epicondyle. There is commonly some peritendinous fluid noted. Power Doppler is often useful in demonstrating marked neovascularization most commonly in the extensor carpi radialis brevis.

## Posterior Elbow

### Distal Triceps Tendon Injury

Acute rupture of the triceps tendon manifests with inability to extend the elbow. When there is a lot of swelling and pain inhibiting the exam, the ultrasound is valuable in demonstrating tendon disruption with wavy appearance of the distal tendon and retraction. Chronic tendinosis may also occur and is manifested with hypoechoic areas in the tendon along with neovascularization seen on power Doppler. One must be careful to not over-interpret the fat that normally sits between the layers of triceps as tendinosis.

### Cubital Tunnel Syndrome

Excessive compression of the ulnar nerve may occur within the proximal cubital groove or the more distal cubital tunnel. This may be secondary to extrinsic compression of the nerve by thickened arcuate ligament, bony spurs, soft-tissue masses such as a lipoma, or a congenital anconeus epitrochlearis. This latter entity is a normal variant in up to one-third of the population and represents a medial anconeus muscle forming the roof of the cubital tunnel, which can act as a space-occupying lesion in the groove. Inflammatory and crystal diseases are also considered.

These patients will present with medial elbow pain and signs of distal nerve compression with paresthesias of the ulnar two fingers and intrinsic muscle wasting. The most common sonographic finding is sudden narrowing of the nerve at the compression site with proximal swelling of the nerve. A cross-sectional area of greater than 7.9 mm$^2$ has been identified as an upper limit of normal for the ulnar nerve. Inflammation around the nerve may also be seen.

### Cubital Instability

The ulnar nerve may sublux out of the cubital groove or frankly dislocate in elbow flexion. This is usually caused by the medial portion of the triceps muscle and can easily be seen with an axial (transverse or short-axis) view of the cubital groove with flexion of the elbow. However, this may be seen in asymptomatic individuals.

### Olecranon Bursitis

The olecranon bursa is dorsal to the olecranon and quite superficial. It is not usually visible unless inflamed or infected. It will readily appear as a hypoechoic fluid collection when enlarged. A thickened wall may appear if chronically inflamed. Local trauma and inflammatory and infectious causes must be considered. Calcific triceps tendinopathy may also cause bursa swelling.

## Red Flags

- When a ruptured distal biceps is suspected, the ultrasound is *not* the definitive imaging method. The angular changes of the distal biceps make it difficult to differentiate anisotropic changes from tendon tears. Furthermore, there are two heads of the biceps insertion, the long and short heads. The long head may not be visible at its deeper attachment to the radial tuberosity.
- When a joint effusion is noted, it is not possible to distinguish an infected from an inflamed effusion. Aspiration may be indicated to make this differentiation. Similarly, an infected olecranon bursa will not have systemic symptoms initially. As such, when there is pain and warmth, an aspiration is critical in the evaluation.
- Avoiding injection into vessels is critical. Particularly when injecting near the deep branch of the radial nerve and the ulnar nerve, use of power Doppler is helpful in identifying the recurrent radial and ulnar arteries.

## Pearls and Pitfalls

- The elbow has many bony prominences that provide sudden changes in tendon direction. As such, the ultrasound beam will suddenly lose its perpendicular alignment with the tendon, and artifact anisotropy is common. This is particularly true of the biceps tendon. It is important to toggle the probe in a heel-to-toe manner with compression gently into the soft tissues distally. This will allow reduction of the anisotropy. The addition of tissue harmonics to the image may also be useful to define the deeper layers of the biceps tendon.
- A common anterior injection is a radial tunnel nerve block. This PIN block is achieved with visualization of the anterior elbow in extension, with varying amounts of supination and pronation depending on the individual patient. An axial (transverse or short-axis) view of the nerve is attained at the supinator muscle over the radial neck. An in-plane approach from lateral to medial is easily achieved with the needle parallel to the probe. It is important to identify and avoid the recurrent radial artery and superficial branch of the radial nerve.
- On the medial aspect, a common injection is the peritendinous area of the common flexor group. Here, the supine patient places the arm in abduction and external rotation with full supination. Varying amounts of elbow flexion are used depending on the patient. A longitudinal (long-axis) view of the tendon is attained on the medial aspect

of the medial epicondyle, which is kept in view. The ulnar nerve and median nerve with brachial artery should have been previously identified and avoided. The approach is from distal to proximal with an in-plane approach. Care is taken to avoid entering the tendon as well as being too superficial if corticosteroids are injected, because they can cause fat atrophy and depigmentation.

- When approaching a peritendinous injection of the common extensor tendon, the supine patient places the elbow in about 40° of flexion with full pronation of the forearm. The image is attained in the longitudinal plane (long axis) just to the volar side of the common extensor tendon over the radial head. An in-plane approach from distal to proximal is performed. The radial nerve and recurrent radial artery should be avoided. Also avoid entering the tendon as well as fat atrophy and depigmentation of the skin.
- The cubital tunnel provides a very narrow area for the probe in a transverse or short-axis view. This will narrow the field of view significantly. To enhance this step, stand-off gel pads may be used for visualization and are available in sterile disposable forms for interventional procedures. Alternatively, copious amounts of gel under the edges will fill the gap for peripheral visualization.
- Dynamic maneuvers may offer tremendous advantages to the elbow examination, but abnormalities do not always indicate pathology. For instance, valgus stress of the elbow imaged medially in about 20° of flexion is a nice technique to demonstrate laxity of the UCL. However, asymptomatic pitchers have demonstrated increased laxity of the medial joint that does not need intervention. This is likely due to chronic stretch to the ligament.
- Similarly, subluxation of the ulnar nerve over the epicondyle may be demonstrated with an axial (transverse or short-axis) view of the cubital tunnel during flexion. Here, the distal triceps may sublux the nerve over the epicondyle or even dislocate over the common flexor tendon. This has been demonstrated in over 15 % of the normal asymptomatic population. However, in unusual cases it may be associated with friction neuritis and demonstrated with focal swelling of the nerve at the area of subluxation. This is best demonstrated on a long-axis view of the nerve.

## Clinical Exercise

Certain "homework assignments" are easily achieved for the elbow. The student can readily examine his or her own non-dominant elbow. In the seated position and facing the ultrasound monitor, the following steps are performed and recorded:

1. The imaging settings are set for the linear array probe for a high frequency (10–17 MHz). The depth is set to a shallow level with a shallow focus.

2. The anterior elbow is visualized in an axial (transverse or short-axis) plane above, at, and below the joint. An image is recorded with identification of the pronator teres, median nerve, brachial artery, brachialis muscle, biceps tendon with muscle, and radial nerve. The probe is then turned longitudinally (long-axis view), and images are taken in the radial and ulnar sagittal views. The technique of changing from a transverse or short-axis to a longitudinal or long-axis view while maintaining a central view of the biceps tendon is practiced. The brachialis and bicep tendons are identified along with the anterior recess. Heel-to-toe toggle on the biceps tendon distally is used to demonstrate anisotropy.

3. The medial elbow is imaged in the longitudinal (long) axis over the UCL and common flexor tendon. The image is recorded with identifying markings of these two structures.

4. The lateral elbow is imaged over the lateral epicondyle in a longitudinal (long) axis view of the common extensor tendon over the lateral epicondyle and radial head. These structures are imaged with identifying markers.

5. The student may demonstrate needle placement in both long- and short-axis views with a pig's foot or phantom gel block. With the pig's foot, tendon injections can be practiced. The student will demonstrate appropriate placement with long- and short-axis views.

## Suggested Reading

Beggs I, Bianchi S, Buenos A, Cohen M, Court-Payen, Grainger A, et al. Musculoskeletal ultrasound technical guidelines II. Elbow. European Society for Musculoskeletal Radiology. http://www.essr.org/html/img/pool/elbow.pdf.

Bianchi S, Martinoli C. Elbow. In: Bianchi S, Martinoli C, editors. Ultrasound of the musculoskeletal system. Berlin: Springer; 2007. p. 349–407.

Thoirs K, Williams M, Phillips M. Systematic review of sono-graphic measurements of the ulnar nerve at the elbow. J Diagn Med Sonog. 2007;23:255–62.

# Shoulder

9

Mark E. Lavallee

## Approach to the Joint

The shoulder is comprised of three bones: the humerus, the clavicle, and the scapula. The shoulder contains four joints: the glenohumeral joint, the acromioclavicular joint, the sternoclavicular joint, and the scapulothoracic joint. The first three joints can be easily visualized by ultrasound. Anterior structures include the long head of the biceps tendon, the subscapularis muscle/tendon, the anterior deltoid, the acromioclavicular capsule, and the coracoid process. The superior structures include the acromioclavicular joint/capsule, the clavicle, the acromion process, and the trapezius. The lateral structures include the deltoid, the subscapularis, the supraspinatus, the subacromial bursa, the joint capsule, and the superior labrum. The posterior aspects of the shoulder include the scapula, the trapezius, the supraspinatus, the infraspinatus/teres minor, the subscapularis, the joint capsule, the suprascapular nerve, the posterior labrum, and the rhomboid muscles.

M.E. Lavallee, M.D., C.S.C.S., F.A.C.S.M. (✉)
South Bend-Notre Dame Sports Medicine Fellowship Program,
South Bend, IN, USA

Department of Family Medicine, Indiana University School
of Medicine, Indianapolis, IN, USA

Memorial Hospital of South Bend and Memorial Medical Group,
South Bend, IN, USA

Indiana University South Bend, South Bend, IN, USA

Holy Cross College, South Bend, IN, USA

University of Notre Dame, Men's Soccer Team,
South Bend, IN, USA

USA Weightlifting, Sports Medicine Society,
Colorado Springs, CO, USA

Division of Sports Medicine, Department of Family Medicine,
Memorial Hospital of South Bend, 111 West Jefferson, Suite 100,
South Bend, IN 46601, USA
e-mail: mlavallee@memorialsb.org

With ultrasound, you can look at these structures both statically and with dynamic motion.

## Probe/Machine Settings

For the shoulder examination, using the linear array probe is recommended. High-frequency linear probes can range from 5 to 15 MHz with frequencies between 7 and 10 MHz best for imaging the rotator cuff.

The shoulder joint requires a specific number of images be captured to be considered a *complete* scan. Anything less than this number will be considered a *limited* scan by most insurance carriers. A complete scan of the shoulder [1] contains the following captured views:

- Long head of bicep tendon (anterior) in bicipital groove (transverse or short and longitudinal or long axis)
- Subscapularis tendon (anterior) external rotation (short and long axis)
- Supraspinatus, biceps tendon, and subscapularis tendon (rotator cuff interval) (anterolateral), also known as the "Marilyn Monroe pose" (long axis)
- Supraspinatus tendon (anterolateral) (short axis)
- Infraspinatus/teres minor (posterior) (long axis)
- Subacromial bursa size
- Acromioclavicular joint (coronal)
- Suprascapular notch (optional)
- Spinoglenoid notch
  Additional imaging that may be done if needed or desired may include:
- Dynamic views of the rotator cuff
- Contralateral shoulder as needed to assess normal

## Common Conditions

The following sections discuss the most common pathologic conditions that lend themselves to visualization using ultrasound.

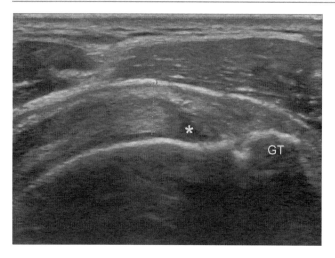

**Fig. 9.1** Partial undersurface tear of supraspinatus (marked with *asterisk*)

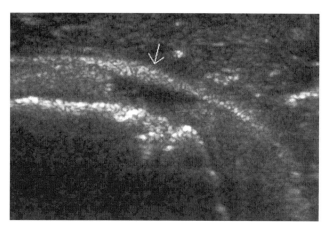

**Fig. 9.2** Complete tear with retraction of supraspinatus

## Partial-Thickness Rotator Cuff Tear

With ultrasound, the examiner should be able to ascertain if the tear is humeral side/inferior side or acromial side/superior side. It is important to view the "critical area," near the insertion of the supraspinatus on the humerus (Fig. 9.1).

## Complete-Thickness Rotator Cuff Tear

Ultrasound will show retraction of tendon. A dynamic evaluation may show this when it is not evident on static examination (Fig. 9.2).

## Calcific Tendonitis

Ultrasound will pick up small calcific areas in the tendon, especially when assessed dynamically. MRI and CT scan can visualize this pathology, if larger than 5 mm. Most symptomatic lesions are 5 mm or less. Plain radiographs also identify these calcifications (Fig. 9.3a, b).

## Biceps Tendonitis/Tenosynovitis

Ultrasound can ascertain between normal tendon vs. diseased (partial/full tears, tendonosis). Short-axis view of proximal biceps tendon will show a hyperechoic "fluid ring" around the tendon if there is fluid in the sheath. Ultrasound is effective at seeing neovascularization, a pathologic condition associated with tendonosis, which MRI, CT, and radiographs aren't able to assess (Fig. 9.4).

## Acromioclavicular Joint Arthropathy

Radiographs are the mainstay for grading acromioclavicular separations and degenerative joint disease. Ultrasound also identifies osteophytes and narrowed joint space; however, it also allows visualization of the "geyser" appearance of a joint effusion and thickened capsule (Fig. 9.5).

## Subacromial Bursitis

Ultrasound is highly sensitive tool to see this structure. It can often be missed on MRI, if sequencing or image cuts are greater than 2 mm (Fig. 9.6).

## Adhesive Capsulitis

A thickened glenohumeral capsule can be seen on anterior and posterior views. Capsular distension via intra-articular injection under ultrasound guidance is often easily accomplished and visualized.

## Biceps Tendon Subluxation

This is rarely diagnosed in static imaging studies like MR or CT, but ultrasound can easily see this dynamically.

## Red Flags

There are some conditions that need urgent attention. These include posterior dislocation of the sternoclavicular joint, as it may compress the internal/external carotids. This is a vascular emergency on many different levels. Vascular ultrasound is beyond the scope of this chapter, but in an emergency situation, the vessels can be imaged quickly via the color flow or Doppler flow setting on the machine. Other emergencies in relation to the shoulder, like glenohumeral dislocation or humeral neck fracture, lend themselves to radiography as the preferred imaging choice. Although sonographic imaging is not preferred, it could be utilized in a situation where radiography and other modalities are not accessible.

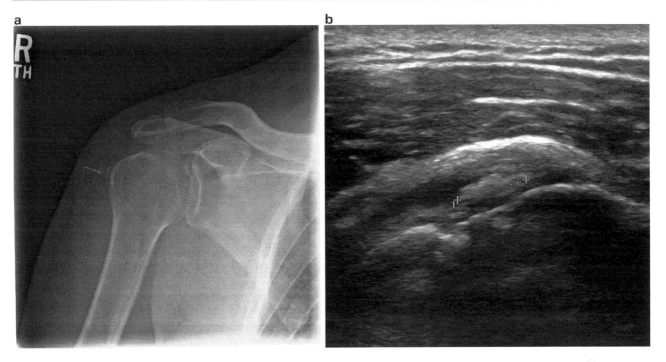

**Fig. 9.3** (**a**, **b**) Calcification in infraspinatus

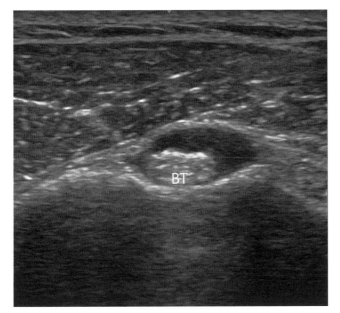

**Fig. 9.4** Increased fluid around biceps tendon (BT), long-axis view

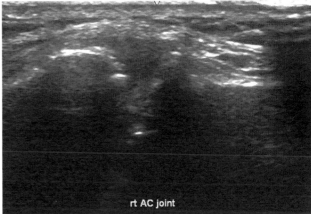

**Fig. 9.5** Acromioclavicular joint with arthropathy

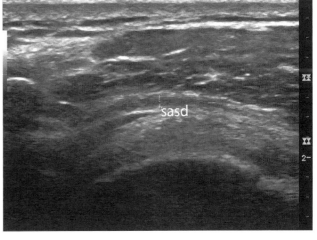

**Fig. 9.6** Subacromial-subdeltoid bursitis (sasd)

Subclavian steal syndrome, brachial artery thrombosis, aneurysm, or dissection are all urgent conditions in the shoulder region that are best imaged via vascular ultrasound, MR, or CT angiography. Do not try to use ultrasound to rule out labral pathology. Though certain aspects of the labrum can be visualized and even labral tears diagnosed, ultrasound does not truly inspect the whole labrum. MRI or MR arthrogram is currently the most sensitive diagnostic imaging for labral tear. It should be mentioned that although ultrasound is excellent at identifying fluid-filled superficial structures (i.e., bursas, hematomas, and joint capsules), the current technology cannot differentiate between different type of fluids. A hemarthrosis and a septic joint will look similar, and one cannot determine whether an enlarged subacromial bursa is infected or just inflamed.

## Pearls and Pitfalls

Here are some common tips that might prove helpful:

### Anisotropy

When looking at the insertion point of a rotator cuff muscle, realize the hypoechoic area at the insertion may not be a tear but anisotropy (echo shadow). This can be delineated by slow activation of the glenohumeral joint or "toggling" the transducer, which will remove the anisotropy.

### Positioning

Getting your patient (and yourself) into a stable and relaxed position is crucial. The patient should be seated on a stool rather than the exam table. The examiner may stand or also be seated on a stool (slightly higher than the patient). Many learners tend to grip the probe too high and too tight, or insist on standing (instead of sitting). Sit down and relax your grip. Position your hand at the distal part of the probe. Allow part of your hand or fingers to rest on the patient for stability.

### Orientation

Every time you place your probe on the patient's skin, orient yourself! Place only one corner of the linear probe on the patient's skin in order to confirm which side of visual field is medial vs. lateral or proximal vs. distal.

### Color Flow

For musculoskeletal conditions, color flow is usually not needed unless looking at vasculature or injecting under ultrasound. Color flow can also be used to ascertain if a structure has neovascularization, a pathologic condition.

### Depth

Adjust the depth of visual field to the lowest allowable in order to see the structures you need to see. This allows a wider viewing area and more resolution.

## Pictographs

Consider using these if available. Pull them in prior to scanning. They will save you lots of editing and typing later.

## Save Images

After capturing still or video clips of structures, do not forget to label and save the image. For a complete shoulder exam, you should have saved around 10–12 images; for a limited scan, 3–6 images. Minimize video clips (make them short, as they can easily take up your memory).

## Become Ambidextrous

Learn to hold the probe and scan with either hand. Also, become comfortable with injecting with either hand.

## Advanced Use of Ultrasound

Certain conditions may render themselves to imaging via ultrasound once a clinician is more experienced; these conditions include distal biceps tendon injury, nerve evaluation, SLAP tears, and anterior glenohumeral labrum.

## Clinical Exercise

1. Shoulder [2] (Table 9.1)

    Homework assignment for reader: Attempt to find these structures when doing the ultrasound exam of the shoulder. In order to perform a "complete" shoulder exam, one will need to be able to capture the images.
    - Biceps tendon (anterior view)
    - Subscapularis (anterior approach)
    - Dynamic examination for biceps tendon subluxation (as indicated)
    - Acromioclavicular joint (anterior and superior views)
    - Infraspinatus (posterior approach)
    - Posterior glenohumeral joint (posterior view)
    - Coracoid process and anterior humeral head (anterior view) approach for anterior intra-articular glenohumeral injection
    - Supraspinatus (short and long axis) and subacromial bursa
    - Dynamic rotator cuff evaluation
    - Spinoglenoid notch (posterior view)
    - Rotator cuff interval: supraspinatus, biceps tendon, and subscapularis ("Marilyn Monroe" shot or "hand in back pocket" shot)

**Table 9.1** Anterior shoulder[a]

| Anatomy | Patient position | Transducer position and description | Picture of scan and labeled structures | Pearls/pitfalls |
|---|---|---|---|---|
| Long head of biceps (proximal) | Patient is seated arm at side, elbow flexed, palm up | 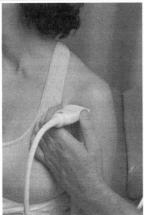<br>Transverse or short-axis view<br>Probe over anterior deltoid, axial to upper arm | 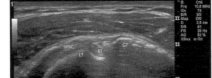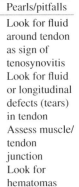<br>Short-axis (axial) image<br>Labeled structures<br>BT—biceps tendon<br>GT—greater tuberosity<br>LT—lesser tuberosity<br>SUSC—subscpularis | Look for fluid around tendon as sign of tenosynovitis<br>Look for fluid or longitudinal defects (tears) in tendon<br>Assess muscle/ tendon junction<br>Look for hematomas |
|  |  | 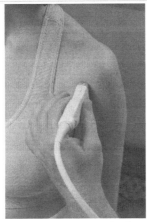<br>Longitudinal or long-axis view<br>Probe over anterior deltoid, longitudinal to upper arm, scan to muscle tendon junction | 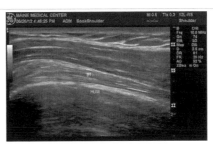<br>Long-axis image<br>Labeled structures<br>BT—biceps tendon<br>HUM—humerus | *Dynamic biceps evaluation*<br>Patient is seated, arm at side. Have patient externally rotate forearm with elbow at side, palm up<br>Look for bicep tendon moving out of the bicipital groove<br>Without this maneuver, a subluxing or dislocating biceps tendon could be overlooked |
|  |  | 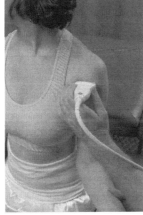<br>Short-axis view<br>Probe over anterior deltoid, axial to upper arm | 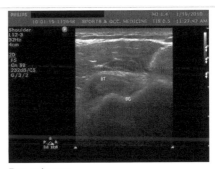<br>Dynamic scan<br>Labeled structures<br>BT—biceps tendon<br>BG—bicipital groove |  |

(continued)

**Table 9.1** (continued)

| Anatomy | Patient position | Transducer position and description | Picture of scan and labeled structures | Pearls/pitfalls |
|---|---|---|---|---|
| Subscapularis tendon | Patient is seated arm at side, elbow flexed, arm externally rotated palm up | 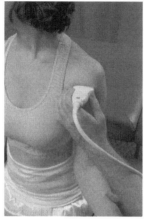<br>Short-axis view<br>Probe over anterior deltoid, axial | 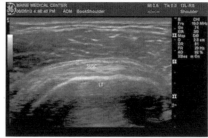<br>Long-axis image<br>Labeled structures<br>LT—lesser tuberosity<br>SUSC—subscapularis | *Note*: Given the orientation of the subscapularis, the longitudinal view is actually a transverse view of the muscle/tendon. Note the dark areas interspersed between the white-appearing tendon fibers—these are areas of muscle tissue |
| | | 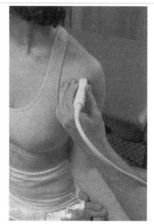<br>Long-axis view<br>Longitudinal to upper arm | 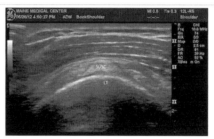<br>Long-axis image<br>Labeled structures<br>LT—lesser tuberosity<br>SUSC—subscapularis | |
| Rotator cuff interval (subscapularis, biceps tendon, supraspinatus) | Patient facing direction of shoulder being studied, 90° to the examiner with hand on "back pocket" and elbow tucked in | 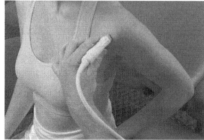<br>Short-axis view<br>Axial over bicipital groove, sweep transducer proximally to the acromion to view supraspinatus; distally down to view infraspinatus | 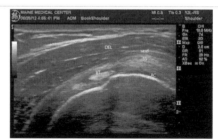<br>Long-axis or "Marilyn Monroe" image<br>Labeled structures<br>DEL—deltoid muscle<br>BT—biceps tendon<br>SS—suprapsinatous<br>AC—articualar cartilage<br>sasd—subacromial-subdeltoid bursa | Supraspinatus can look like a "tire on a wheel"<br>This position shows the "rotator cuff interval"; same location of proximal biceps tendon<br>Note that the noninflamed subacromial-subdeltoid bursa appears as a thin, dark line between the supraspinatus and deltoid |

(continued)

**Table 9.1** (continued)

| Anatomy | Patient position | Transducer position and description | Picture of scan and labeled structures | Pearls/pitfalls |
|---|---|---|---|---|
| | | 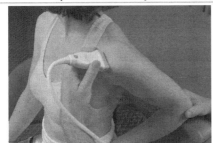<br>Long-axis view<br>Relocate bicipital groove and identify footprint of supraspinatus | 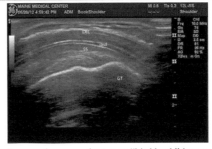<br>Long-axis supraspinatus or "bird beak" image<br>Labeled structures<br>DEL—deltoid<br>sasd—subacromial-subdeltoid bursa<br>SS—supraspinatus<br>GT—greater tuberosity | Supraspinatus looks like a "bird beak" Notice that the superficial aspect of the supraspinatus should bulge or be convex If concave or "dented," may indicate a tear Bright (hyperechoic) cartilage signal may indicate a tear Make sure to evaluate "criticalzone"—insertion of supraspinatus |
| Anterior glenohumeral joint and coracoid process | Patient is seated arm at side, elbow flexed, palm up | 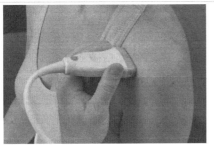<br>Short-axis view<br>Probe over anterior deltoid and coracoid process, axial to upper arm | 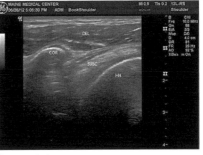<br>Long-axis image<br>Labeled structures<br>COR—coronoid process<br>DEL—deltoid<br>SUSC—subscapularis<br>HH—humeral head | Preferred approach for anterior glenohumeral injection Can often visualize a portion of superior labrum |

ᵃTransducer is a 3- to 15-MHz probe. The patient is seated on a stool, and the examiner is seated on a stool or standing

2. Anterior shoulder
   - Identify biceps tendon and bicipital groove of humerus.
   - Attempt a dynamic examination of the proximal biceps tendon to attempt to sublux it. Capture video clip while flexing elbow with resisted external rotation at shoulder.
   - Identify subscapularis (arm externally rotated). Identify the supraspinatus, biceps tendon, and subscapularis, all in one image. Rotator cuff interval or "Marilyn Monroe" shot.
   - Identify coracoid process and humeral head in same image (anterior injection portal).
   - Dynamic view of the anterior shoulder during internal and external rotation. *Note*: appearance of subscapularis with external rotation and then appearance of supraspinatus with internal rotation.

3. Superior shoulder (Table 9.2)
   - Identify the acromioclavicular joint.
4. Lateral shoulder
   - Identify supraspinatus as it inserts on the humeral head (short- and long-axis views) (posterolateral portal for subacromial injection).
   - Identify subacromial bursa. Measure with calipers its length, height, and circumference.
   - Dynamically visualize supraspinatus when shoulder is abducted. Look for impingement.
5. Posterior shoulder (Table 9.3)
   - Identify infraspinatus, as it inserts onto humeral head.
   - Identify posterior glenohumeral joint capsule and labrum (posterior portal for subacromial injection).
   - Identify the spinoglenoid notch, deep to infraspinatus.

**Table 9.2** Superior and lateral shoulder[a]

| Anatomy | Patient position | Transducer position and description | Picture of scan and labeled structures | Pearls/pitfalls |
|---|---|---|---|---|
| Superior acromio-clavicular joint | Patient is seated, arm at side, elbow relaxed, palm up | Long axis over distal clavicle | Labeled structures ACJ—acromioclavicular joint JC—joint capsule ACR—acromion CL—clavicle | Sweep probe over joint both anterior and posterior Thickened capsule, narrowed joint space, osteophytes indicate a degenerative joint Increase fluid in joint capsule or "Geyser sign" could indicate recent trauma, rheumatologic issues, etc. May inject short axis or longitudinally |
| | Dynamic, longitudinal. Same position as above. Hold probe while having the patient abduct the shoulder while keeping the arm internally rotated | Dynamic, long axis | Image of supraspinatus impinging Labeled structures ACR—acromion SS—supraspinatus GT—greater tuberosity | Differential diagnosis should include adhesive capsulitis, impingement, partial tear, and subacromial bursitis |

[a]Transducer is a 3- to 15-MHz probe. The patient is seated on a stool, and the examiner is seated on a stool or standing

**Table 9.3** Posterior shoulder table[a]

| Anatomy | Patient position | Transducer position and description | Picture of scan and labeled structures | Pearls/pitfalls |
|---|---|---|---|---|
| Infraspinatus | Patient is seated, back toward examiner, arm at side, elbow relaxed; probe place longitudinally of posterior glenohumeral joint | Long axis to glenohumeral joint | Labeled structures: IS—infraspinatous HH—humeral head | Scanning superior above scapular spine visualizes the supraspinatus muscle. Below the spine, the infraspinatus and teres minor are seen Suprascapular notch may have a cyst present |

(continued)

**Table 9.3**  (continued)

| Anatomy | Patient position | Transducer position and description | Picture of scan and labeled structures | Pearls/pitfalls |
|---|---|---|---|---|
| Spinoglenoid notch | As above | As above. Slide transducer slightly medially to visualize spinoglenoid notch | <br>Labeled structures:<br>HH—humeral head<br>L—labrum<br>G—glenoid<br>SNG—spinoglenoid notch<br>IS—infraspinatous | Posterior capsule can be seen for glenohumeral joint injection<br>Preferred posterior approach for glenohumeral joint injections |
| Teres minor | As above | Slide slightly distally to visualize teres minor | <br>Labeled structures:<br>H—humerus<br>TM—teres minor | |

[a]Transducer is a 3- to 15-MHz probe. The patient is seated on a stool, and the examiner is seated on a high stool or standing

# References

1. American Institute of Ultrasound in Medicine. AIUM practice guideline for the performance of a shoulder ultrasound examination. J Ultrasound Med. 2003;22(10):1137–41.
2. Finnoff J, Lavallee M, Smith J. Musculoskeletal ultrasound education for sports medicine fellows: a suggested/potential curriculum by the American Medical Society for Sports Medicine. Br J Sports Med. 2010;44(16):1144–50.

# Suggested Reading

Beggs I, Bianchi S, Bueno A, Cohen M, Court-Payen M, Grainger A, et al. Musculoskeletal ultrasound technical guidelines. I. The shoulder. European Society of Musculoskeletal Radiology http://www.essr.org/html/img/pool/shoulder.pdf.

Hill J, Lavallee M. Musculoskeletal ultrasonography. In: Pfenniger JL, Fowler GS, editors. Pfenniger and Fowler's procedures in primary care. 3rd ed. New York: Elsevier; 2011. p. 1233–45.

McNally E. Practical musculoskeletal ultrasound. New York: Churchill Livingstone; 2005.

# Foo and Toes

## Kevin deWeber

## Approach to the Joint

To image the foot and toes most efficiently, the examiner should be seated on a stool at the end of the table facing the patient with legs extended toward the examiner. The ultrasound machine should be placed directly adjacent to either side of the table for ease of viewing.

The patient should lie on the table. The patient may need to be supine, prone, or in a lateral side-lying position, depending on the structure to be imaged. As a rule, place the area to be imaged facing upward or toward the examiner.

## Probe Selection

Use a linear transducer with medium to high frequency, which should include 12 MHz, and preferably higher for imaging of toes. Use of a padded "standoff" probe cover or a thick layer of gel may be needed to accommodate the bony contours of the toes. If available, a "hockey stick"-shaped probe allows easier access to tight areas.

## Specific Presets

These are the same as for hand and fingers—usually a shallow depth (2–3 cm)—and as high a frequency as your probe will allow.

K. deWeber, MD, FAAFP, FACSM, RMSK (✉)
Department of Family Medicine, Uniformed Services
University of the Health Sciences, 4301 Jones Bridge Road, Bethesda,
MD 20814, USA
e-mail: kdsportsmd@gmail.com

## Common Problems

Interdigital neuromas, plantar fasciopathy, sinus tarsi syndrome, and inflammatory arthritides are the most common conditions in the foot amenable to examination and intervention using ultrasound. Less common conditions include entrapments of the medial and lateral plantar nerves and medial calcaneal nerve, fractures of the metatarsal shafts, and midfoot sprains (Lisfranc). Ultrasound-guided sinus tarsi injection and aspiration of the metatarsophalangeal and subtalar joints for synovial fluid analysis in suspected arthritis are likely to be more accurate than landmark-guided procedures (Table 10.1).

## Pitfalls and Red Flags

- Subtalar joint injections: both the anterolateral and posterolateral approaches have been shown in cadaver studies to be safe and highly accurate. The anterolateral approach affords the shortest needle path but requires a short-axis approach, while the posterolateral approach affords an in-plane longitudinal needle guidance but at a greater depth and steep angle. Do not attempt to penetrate the subtalar joint from a posteromedial approach. The posterior tibial artery and veins and the tibial nerve are immediately overlying the joint and can easily be injured [1, 2].
- Interdigital space: be careful to differentiate an interdigital neuroma, which will have a fusiform shape continuous with the interdigital nerve, from an interdigital bursa, which lies more dorsally in the interspace.

## Pearls

- While ultrasound is useful to determine whether the subtalar joint or a digital joint has an effusion, this cannot distinguish between infection and inflammatory arthritis. Obtaining fluid for analysis will usually be necessary.

**Table 10.1** Foot and toes

| Patient position | Transducer position and description | Picture of scan and labeled structures | Pearls/pitfalls |
|---|---|---|---|
| Patient supine, knee bent 90°, sole of foot resting flat on table | 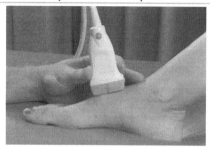<br>Longitudinal (or long) axis to foot<br>Midfoot at tarso-metatarsal joints | 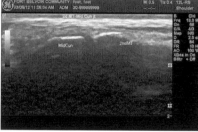<br>Labeled structures<br>MidCun—middle cuneiform<br>MT—metatarsal | In midfoot sprains, do weight-bearing images of both affected and normal feet to determine if there is any widening or step-offs of any tarso-metatarsal joints. Weight-bearing X-rays are necessary also. Any fractures or widening between bones may require surgical correction |
| Same as above | 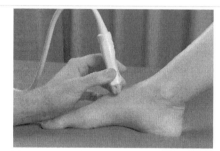<br>Transverse or short axis to foot<br>Midfoot at proximal intermetatarsal spaces | 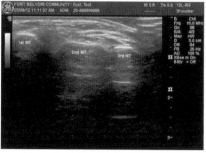<br>Labeled structures<br>MT—metatarsal | Same as above |
| Patient lying on affected side, lateral aspect of affected foot resting on table, medial foot facing upward | 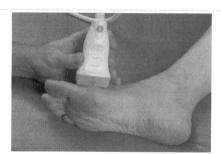<br>Long axis to first MTP joint, medially or dorsally | 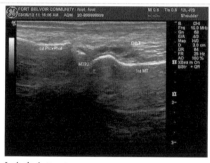<br>Labeled structures<br>Prox Phal—proximal phalanx<br>MT—metatarsal<br>MTPJ—metatarsophalangeal joint<br>EHLT—extensor hallucis longus tendon | Good location to obtain fluid from first MTP joint. Access the joint space medial to the EHL (extensor hallucis longus) tendon or on the medial joint space. Enter with needle in short axis to transducer |
| Patient lying on affected side, lateral aspect of affected foot resting on table, medial foot facing upward, or may be done with patient prone | 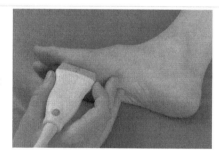<br>Long axis to first MTP joint, plantar | 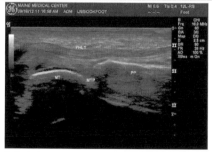<br>Labeled structures<br>FHLT—flexor hallucis longus tendon<br>MT—metatarsal<br>MTP—metatarsophalangeal joint<br>PP—proximal phalanx | |

(continued)

**Table 10.1**   (continued)

| Patient position | Transducer position and description | Picture of scan and labeled structures | Pearls/pitfalls |
|---|---|---|---|
| Patient lying on affected side, lateral aspect of affected foot resting on table, medial foot facing upward, or may be done with patient prone | 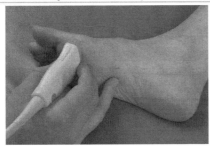<br>Sesamoids<br>Short axis to first MTP joint, plantar | 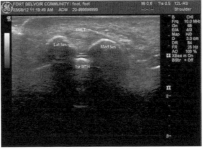<br>Labeled structures<br>FHLT—flexor hallucis longus tendon<br>Med/Lat Ses—medial and lateral sesamoids<br>MTH—metatarsal head | |
| As above, now with finger dorsal, interdigital; apply gentle pressure | 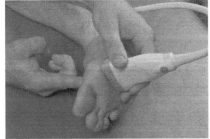<br>Interdigital neuroma<br>Short axis over affected interdigital space | 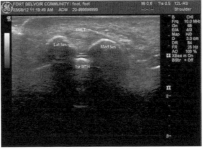<br>Labeled structures<br>MTH—metatarsal head<br>3/4 Inter MTH—intermetatarsal space between third and fourth metatarsals | Place your finger on dorsal aspect of foot in affected interdigital space and compress tissue between probe and finger to reproduce symptoms and confirm location of neuroma |
| Same as above | 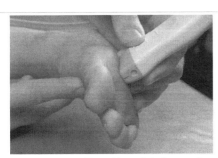<br>Long axis over affected interdigital space for neuroma | 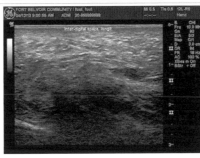<br>Labeled structures<br>IDS—interdigital space | Fairly unremarkable looking when normal. Neuroma may appear as a fusiform hypoechoic thickening of the nerve |
| Patient prone, foot hanging off edge of table | 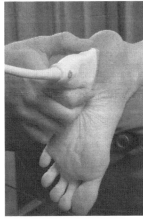<br>Long axis to foot<br>Plantar fascia, long axis | 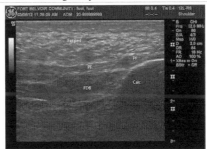<br>Labeled structures<br>PF—plantar fascia<br>FDB—flexor digitorum brevis<br>Calc—calcaneus | Keep the ankle at a neutral angle to avoid loosening the plantar fascia and giving it a wavy, irregular appearance |

(continued)

**Table 10.1** (continued)

| Patient position | Transducer position and description | Picture of scan and labeled structures | Pearls/pitfalls |
|---|---|---|---|
| Alternate: foot on table with rolled towel under ankle, keeping ankle joint near neutral | 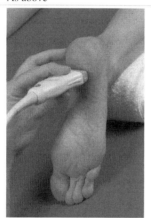<br>As above | 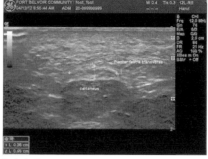<br>Labeled structures<br>Calc—calcaneus | |
| Same as above | 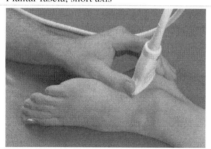<br>Short axis to foot<br>Plantar fascia, short axis | <br>Labeled structures<br>Calc—calcaneus<br>ST—sinus tarsi | With short-axis slides, image the proximal 1–2 cm of the fascia, where most plantar fasciopathy occurs. Look for hypoechoic swelling. This is a good approach for guiding a needle into the affected fascia. Enter heel medially with needle |
| Patient prone, hip slightly flexed and externally rotated, and knee slightly bent, with medial aspect of foot resting on table and lateral foot up | 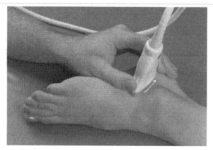<br>Sinus tarsi<br>Short to long axis of the foot just anterior to the lateral malleolus | <br>Labeled structures<br>Calc—calcaneus<br>STJ—subtalar joint<br>PTs—peroneal tendons | Talar neck and anterior process of the calcaneus form the sides of the deep, U-shaped sinus tarsi. Injections can be done with this view using a short-axis approach with a needle angled steeply downward to reach the deep subtalar ligaments that usually cause pain here |
| Same as above | 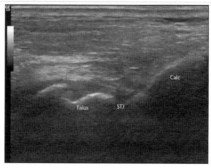<br>Subtalar joint, anterolateral<br>Slide transducer from above location slightly posterior (toward heel) and distal (toward sole) | <br>Labeled structures<br>Talus<br>Calc—calcaneus<br>STJ—subtalar joint | Subtalar (talocalcaneal) joint is narrow and is located just cranially to the peroneal tendons, which are seen in cross-section. If aspirating fluid from this location using short-axis technique, take care to avoid the peroneal tendons and sural nerve, which are usually located caudal to the subtalar joint in this area |

**Table 10.1** (continued)

| Patient position | Transducer position and description | Picture of scan and labeled structures | Pearls/pitfalls |
|---|---|---|---|
| Alternate subtalar joint approach: patient prone or kneeling, leg straight, foot hanging off end of table | 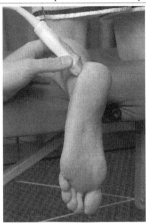<br><br>Subtalar joint, posterolateral. Lateral to Achilles tendon, angle probe slightly medially and caudally | 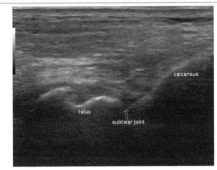 | Examiner's knee can passively dorsiflex the ankle to better visualize the joint space. Using a thick gel layer and light pressure may be necessary to accommodate the patient's contours; a short probe is also helpful. A long-axis needle approach can be used here to access the joint for injections or aspirations |

- Using an ultrasound to guide sinus tarsi injections is well worth the effort. According to a cadaver study, the accuracy of ultrasound-guided sinus tarsi injections is 90 %, while that of non-guided injection is only 35 % [3].

upward. Place the transducer in the long axis just anterior to the lateral malleolus. Identify the sinus tarsi. Then move the transducer posteriorly toward the heel and distally toward the sole. Identify the subtalar joint. Record an image of these structures.

## Clinical Exercise

1. Using your probe on the plantar aspect of the forefoot, identify two adjacent metatarsal heads. Note the interdigital nerve between them. With your other hand, compress the space between the selected metatarsals and observe the nerve being compressed. This is the most common location for interdigital neuromas to occur. They appear as fusiform areas of swelling along the nerve. Record a dynamic evaluation and compression of this area.
2. Have the patient lie in the prone position with the foot to be studied externally rotated so the lateral ankle is facing

## References

1. Henning T, Finoff JT, Smith J. Sonographically guided posterior subtalar joint injections: anatomic study and validation of 3 approaches. PM R. 2009;1:925–31.
2. Smith J, Finoff JT, Henning PT, Turner NS. Accuracy of sonographically guided posterior subtalar joint injections: comparison of 3 techniques. J Ultrasound Med. 2009;28:1549–57.
3. Wisniewski SJ, Smith J, Patterson DG, Carmichael SW, Pawlina W. Ultrasound-guided versus nonguided tibiotalar joint and sinus tarsi injections: a cadaveric study. PM R. 2010;2:277–81.

# Ankle

## John Hatzenbuehler

## Approach to the Joint

The ankle can be a difficult joint to examine using musculoskeletal ultrasound because of the small area and large number of anatomic structures. Using a systematic approach to examining the ankle can be helpful. The ankle is typically divided into four separate quadrants: anterior, medial, lateral, and posterior. Initially, the patient should be positioned supine on a table with the knee flexed to allow the plantar surface of the foot to rest flat on the table. This allows easy access to the anterior quadrant. The examiner should be seated on a stool with rollers at the end of the table to easily facilitate movement from the medial to lateral sides of the ankle. Alternatively, while the patient is supine (on back), the leg may be straightened to allow free motion of the ankle. This will allow the examiner to easily manipulate the ankle and allow for active dorsal and plantar flexion to examine dynamic structures and joint mobility. Occasionally, it may be helpful to lay the patient in the lateral decubitus position with the non-examined leg flexed out of the way to gain easier access to the lateral or medial quadrants. Placing a small pillow or towel on the opposite side of the ankle that is being scanned may help improve probe contact with the skin. The posterior quadrant of the ankle is best examined with the patient lying in the prone (on stomach) position and the ankle lying just off the edge of the table.

## Probe Selection

The ankle joint is one of the more technically difficult joints to ultrasound due to the numerous bony prominences and uneven surfaces. Linear probes with between 7.5- and

J. Hatzenbuehler, M.D. (✉)
Department of Family Medicine, Maine Medical Center,
272 Congress Street, Portland, ME 04103, USA
e-mail: hatzej@mmc.org

15-MHz frequencies are the most useful, as higher frequencies improve superficial structure visualization. Ample use of ultrasound gel is also helpful to allow for full contact of the probe with the uneven ankle structures. Curvilinear probes are generally not recommended because of the superficial nature of the anatomic structures in the ankle.

## Specific Presets

The ultrasound machine should be set to a resolution that best identifies superficial structures. The use of color Doppler is also recommended to help identify the numerous vascular structures present around the ankle.

## Common Problems

Common injuries or musculoskeletal disorders of the ankle are generally identifiable using musculoskeletal ultrasound. Ligament sprains, tendon rupture, peritendinous swelling, joint effusions, and soft-tissue masses are some of the most common indications for using ultrasound.

## Anterior

This quadrant is the best to assess the anterior tendons, such as the tibialis anterior and extensor digitorum and hallucis longus tendons, which are susceptible to overuse injury. The anterior joint line is also easily visible, allowing for identification of an ankle effusion. It is possible to access the joint for injection or aspiration. With slight inversion of the ankle and scanning from the anterior quadrant to the lateral quadrant, the anterior talofibular ligament (ATFL) can be identified; this ligament is commonly injured in inversion ankle sprains. Once identified, a dynamic scan of the ATFL tendon while performing the anterior drawer test can help identify ligament laxity and integrity. This is best

J.M. Daniels and W.W. Dexter (eds.), *Basics of Musculoskeletal Ultrasound*,
DOI 10.1007/978-1-4614-3215-9_11, © Springer Science+Business Media New York 2013

accomplished with the patient lying supine and the ankle positioned just off the end of the table. The probe can be secured with one hand squeezing the tibia and the free hand pulling anterior force on the calcaneus. The use of an assistant is also acceptable to perform this maneuver. See Table 11.1.

## Lateral

When scanning from the anterior quadrant to the lateral quadrant, the ATFL can be visualized. An oblique probe position may be necessary to completely visualize the length of this ligament. An anterior draw test can help evaluate for laxity in this position. The calcaneofibular (CFL) ligament lies just distal to the lateral malleolus and can be visualized by positioning the transducer between the lateral malleolus and calcaneus. Excessive inversion of the ankle will produce a talar tilt test and can help identify the integrity or laxity of the CFL. Posterior to the lateral malleolus, the peroneus brevis and longus tendons can be identified best in the axial plane. Just as with the medial tendons, these lateral tendons are also susceptible to acute tears and overuse injuries. Fluid surrounding the tendons should be visible in these cases. Subluxation of these tendons may also occur, and dynamic ultrasound evaluation is the best way to identify this condition. With the probe secured on the tip of the lateral malleolus and directed posteriorly, the patient can either actively dorsiflex and evert the ankle or the examiner can resist dorsiflexion and eversion motion to see if the peroneal tendons subluxate anteriorly over the lateral malleolus. See Table 11.2.

## Medial

The medial tendon group, which comprises the posterior tibial and flexor digitorum and hallucis longus tendons, is located in this quadrant. Identification of these structures begins in an axial plane (a transverse or short-axis view) with the probe just posterior to the medial malleolus. These tendons can be examined in both the transverse or short-axis and longitudinal or long-axis planes. These tendons are susceptible to acute injury with partial or complete rupture or overuse injury that can cause peritendinous swelling. All of these conditions can be identified using ultrasound scanning.

This is also the location of the tarsal tunnel, where the tibial nerve lies between the more anterior flexor digitorum longus (FDL) tendon and more posterior flexor hallucis longus (FHL) tendon. A palpable prominence on the talus, the sustentaculum tali, is an excellent landmark that can be used to identify the FHC and the tibial nerve, which lies inferiorly to it. The posterior tibial artery (head) and veins (ears) resem-

ble "Mickey Mouse" when viewed on the ultrasound monitor. The tibial nerve can become entrapped in the retinaculum that overlies this tarsal tunnel, commonly causing medial foot and heel pain and numbness. Given the superficial location of the nerve in this area, a hydrodissection procedure can be performed here that can potentially cure tarsal tunnel symptoms. The use of ultrasound for this procedure is critically important, because the posterior tibial artery and vein also lie within the tarsal tunnel and are susceptible to injury with a blind injection. See Table 11.3.

## Posterior

The posterior quadrant is best visualized with the patient lying prone and both feet hanging off the end of the table. This will allow active, unrestricted motion of the ankle and easy comparison view of the other ankle. The Achilles tendon and retrocalcaneal bursa are visualized in this quadrant. Start with the probe in a longitudinal or long-axis orientation and scan the Achilles tendon from the myotendinous junction down to its insertion on the calcaneus. Passive dorsal and plantar flexion of the ankle will give dynamic views of the Achilles tendon to help identify partial- or full-thickness tears. Orienting the probe in the short-axis plane will provide the opportunity to measure Achilles tendon thickness, which can be present in chronic tendinosis. Using the power Doppler setting in either the short- or long-axis planes in areas of thickened Achilles tendon may show neovascularization, which occurs in chronic Achilles tendinopathy. Ultrasound is the best way to visualize the presence of neovascularization. The retrocalcaneal bursa can be visualized in the long-axis plane between the Achilles and the calcaneus, and excess fluid may be visualized in cases of active bursitis. See Table 11.4.

## Red Flags

Ultrasound of the ankle is very helpful to identify fluid in the ankle joint and around tendons. That being said, it is unlikely to be able to differentiate between benign synovitis or tenosynovitis, gouty inflammation, and an infected joint. Ultrasound guidance can be used, however, to help aspirate any ankle effusion for synovial fluid analysis.

Given the numerous tendons around the ankle that are susceptible to injury, complete tears of tendons are possible in each quadrant. Any suspicion for complete tendon tear, especially the Achilles tendon, warrants a high clinical suspicion and thorough clinical exam. The majority of complete tendon ruptures require surgical evaluation. The plantaris tendon is an anatomic variant not present in all patients and can be confused with an intact Achilles tendon in cases of complete Achilles tendon tear. Passive dorsal and plantar

**Table 11.1** The ankle: anterior

| Patient position | Transducer position and description | Picture of scan and labeled structures | Pitfalls/pearls |
|---|---|---|---|
| Patient supine with knees bent and foot flat on table | <br>Transverse or short-axis view<br>Short-axis orientation over anterior ankle<br>Scan proximally to muscle tendon junction | <br>Labeled structures<br>TA—tibialis anterior<br>EDL—extensor digitorum longus<br>EHL—extensor hallucis longus<br>Talus | Find foot extensor tendons<br>Observe flexor tendon fluid $= \dfrac{\text{Tendon tear}}{\text{Tenosynovitis}}$ |
| Patient supine with foot flat on table | <br>Longitudinal or long-axis view<br>Long-axis orientation over anterior ankle<br>Scan length of joint in anterior plane | <br>Labeled structures<br>Tibia<br>Joint rec: anterior joint recess<br>Talar dome | Passively plantarflex and dorsiflex the ankle to indentify joint motion<br>Identify distal tibia, ankle joint, talar dome<br>Effusions and osteophytes are well seen in this view if present |
| Anterior lateral<br>Foot flat on table can have patient slightly invert the ankle | <br>Long-axis view<br>Obliquely oriented probe from lateral malleolus toward talus<br>Move transducer to the anterior tip of distal lateral malleolus<br>Scan length of ligament | <br>Labeled structures<br>LM—lateral malleolus<br>ATFL—anterior talofibular ligament<br>Talus | Identify anterior talofibular ligament (ATFL)<br>Orient the probe obliquely off the lateral malleolus to get full ligament in view<br>With patient lying supine and ankle off table, perform the anterior drawer test with ATFL in view to identify laxity/integrity |

**Table 11.2** The ankle: lateral

| Patient position | Transducer position and description | Picture of scan and labeled structures | Pitfalls/pearls |
|---|---|---|---|
| Either foot flat on table with eversion or patient lying in lateral decubitus position. Keep patient with ankle inverted or lay patient in lateral decubitus with pillow under medial side of ankle | 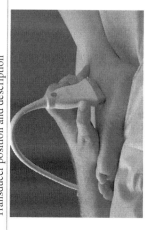<br>Long-axis view<br>Long axis starting at lateral malleolus | 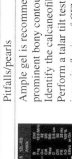<br>Labeled structures<br>LM—lateral malleolus<br>CFL—calcaneofibular ligament<br>Calc—calcaneus | Ample gel is recommended due to prominent bony contours<br>Identify the calcaneofibular ligament (CFL)<br>Perform a talar tilt test to assess for integrity/laxity of CFL |
| Either foot flat on table with eversion or patient lying in lateral decubitus position | 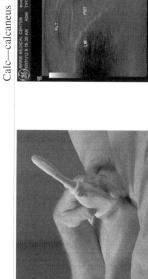<br>Short-axis view<br>Probe behind lateral malleolus<br>Start either posterior to the lateral malleolus or more distally over the lateral calcaneus<br>Scan proximally to identify muscle tendon junction<br>Scan distally to insertion of peroneus brevis on base of 5th metatarsal | 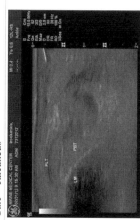<br>Labeled structures<br>LM—lateral malleolus<br>PBT—peroneus brevis tendon<br>PLT—peroneus longus tendon | Observe flexor tendon fluid = $\dfrac{\text{Tendon tear}}{\text{Tenosynovitis}}$<br>Resist ankle eversion and dorsiflexion to identify subluxation if present |

**Table 11.3** The ankle: medial

| Patient position | Transducer position and description | Picture of scan and labeled structures | Pitfalls/pearls |
|---|---|---|---|
| Either patient lying supine with foot flat on table with inversion or patient lying in lateral decubitus position with ankle rotated laterally | <br><br>Short-axis view<br>Probe posterior to medial malleolus<br>Scan proximally to identify muscle tendon junction | <br><br>Labeled structures<br>MM—medial malleolus<br>TP—tibialis posterior tendon<br>FDL—flexor digitorum longus tendon<br>PTA—posterior tibialis artery and (PTV) veins | A small pillow under the lateral ankle may enhance medial structure visualization<br><br>Observe flexor tendon fluid = $\dfrac{\text{Tendon tear}}{\text{Tenosynovitis}}$<br><br>Have the patient flex the toes to distinguish TP from FDL tendons |
| Either foot flat on table with inversion or patient lying in lateral decubitus position | <br><br>Probe oriented anterior and inferior to medial malleolus<br>Sweep transducer around medial malleolus to identify the sustentaculum tali | <br><br>Labeled structures<br>ST—sustentaculum tali<br>FHL—flexor hallucis longus<br>PTN—posterior tibial nerve<br>TA/V—tibial artery and veins | Have patient flex great toe to identify FHL tendon and any peritendinous fluid<br><br>The tibial artery and veins can look like "Mickey Mouse"<br>Tibial nerve will have a speckled-egg appearance |

**Table 11.4** The ankle: posterior

| | | |
|---|---|---|
| Patient prone with foot off the end of the exam table | | Identify the retrocalcaneal bursa |
| | 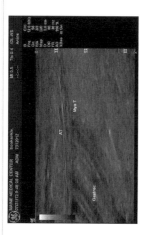 | Passively dorsal and plantar flex the ankle to examine for tears of the Achilles tendon |
| | Labeled structures | Use power Doppler setting over areas of thickened tendon to look for neovascularization |
| | Proximal view | |
| | Gastroc—gastrocnemius muscle | Assess for excess fluid in retrocalcaneal bursa seen in active bursitis |
| | AT—Achilles tendon | |
| | MyoT—myotendinous junction | |
| 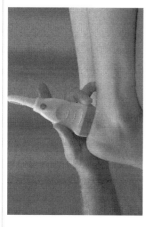 | 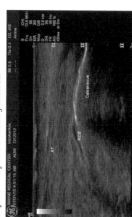 | |
| Long-axis view | Distal view | |
| Long-axis position over Achilles | AT—Achilles tendon | |
| Scan proximally to identify the myotendinous junction and distally to the insertion on the calcaneus | RCB—retrocalcaneal bursa calcaneous | |
| Patient prone with foot off the table | | Measure the size of the Achilles tendon and compare to the other side |
| | 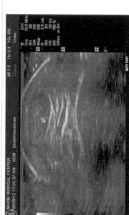 | Neovascularization can be seen in this view as well |
| | | Partial tears are best seen in this view |
|  | Labeled structures | |
| Short-axis view | AT—Achilles tendon | |
| Short-axis position over Achilles | | |
| Scan from myotendinous junction to insertion on calcaneus | | |

flexion of the ankle can help identify partial from complete Achilles tendon tears. Toggling the probe during evaluation of each tendon to resolve anisotropy is helpful to distinguish the presence of partial tendon tears as well.

## Pearls and Pitfalls

The majority of the anatomic structures in the ankle are very superficial in nature. Adjusting the depth and beam penetration resolution to best optimize superficial structures is highly recommended. Also, using ample ultrasound gel to allow for complete contact of the ultrasound probe and the ankle structures will help maximize visualization. Inverting and everting the ankle to flatten out the lateral and medial sides of the ankle, respectively, will also aid in visualization.

Most of the anatomic structures in the ankle are close together. Solid anatomic knowledge of the ankle is necessary to help identify specific structures. Having an anatomy book with labeled structures nearby during the ultrasound examination of the ankle is recommended. Also, dynamic active contraction of muscles can help isolate tendons and distinguish between nearby static structures. Again, strong knowledge of anatomy is helpful in this setting.

The presence of anisotropy in tendons can be both helpful and harmful during ultrasound evaluation of the ankle. The presence of anisotropy in the tendons of the medial ankle, for example, can be used to distinguish the posterior tibial tendon from the posterior tibial vascular structures that are not anisotropic. That being said, tendon anisotropy can be commonly confused with partial tendon tears. Frequent toggling of the probe in areas of hypoechogenicity in tendons can help distinguish partial tears form anisotropy.

## Clinical Exercise

1. In the anterior quadrant, identify the tibialis anterior and extensor hallucis longus tendons by actively resisting ankle dorsiflexion and great to extension, respectively.

2. Identify the ankle joint and passively dorsal and plantar flex the ankle to demonstrate tibial-talar motion.
3. Scan toward the lateral quadrant and identify the ATFL. Perform an anterior drawer test with the ultrasound probe in place to examine for laxity.
4. In the lateral quadrant, identify the peroneal tendons and scan the peroneus brevis tendon down to its insertion on the base of the fifth metatarsal.
5. Resist active eversion of the ankle to assess for peroneal subluxation.
6. In the medial quadrant, actively resist great to flexion to distinguish the FHL from the posterior tibialis tendon.
7. Scan inferior to the medial malleolus to identify the "Mickey Mouse" appearance of the posterior tibial artery and veins.
8. Locate the tibial nerve with its speckled-egg appearance.
9. In the posterior quadrant, scan the length of the Achilles tendon in the long-axis plane from the myotendinous junction to the insertion on the calcaneus.
10. In the short-axis plane, measure the area of the Achilles tendon and compare to the contralateral side.
11. Passively dorsal and plantar flex the ankle to examine the integrity of the Achilles tendon.
12. Use power Doppler mode to examine for neovascularization of the Achilles tendon in both the long- and short-axis planes.

## Suggested Reading

AIUM practice guideline for the performance of the musculoskeletal ultrasound examination; 2007. http://www.aium.org.

Blankenbaker DG, De Smet AA. The role of ultrasound in the evaluation of sports injuries of the lower extremities. Clin Sports Med. 2006;25(4):867–97.

Lin J, Fessell DP, Jacobsen JA, Weadock WJ, Hayes CW. An illustrated tutorial of musculoskeletal sonography: part 3, the lower extremity. Am J Roentgenol. 2000;175(5):1313–21.

Micu MC, Nestrova R, Petranova T, Porta F, Radunovic G, Vlad V, et al. Ultrasound of the ankle and foot in rheumatology. Med Ultrason. 2012;14(1):34–41.

Rogers CJ, Cianca J. Musculoskeletal ultrasound of the ankle and foot. Phys Med Rehabil Clin N Am. 2010;21(3):549–57.

# Knee

Patrick A. Smith and Matt E. Thornburg

## Approach to the Joint

The knee ultrasound exam is carried out after a thorough and systematic history and physical examination. Correlating the patient's complaints of pain and location with focal examination tenderness enhances the potential diagnostic benefit of ultrasound about the knee. Additional important objective evidence of ligamentous laxity can be obtained with dynamic stress ultrasound relative to medial and/or lateral stability. It is best to evaluate the knee systematically beginning anteriorly, then progressing to the medial side, then laterally, and, finally, posteriorly.

## Anterior Knee

The patient is placed in a supine position with the knee in 20–30° of flexion. You may place a pillow under the knee to gain this position and limit anisotropy.

The examiner should sit on a rolling stool on the same side as the effected knee or sit on the edge of the table and have the ultrasound machine across the table.

Longitudinal or long-axis images of the quadriceps tendon are obtained trying to identify the three layers of the tendon, the superficial layer of the rectus femoris, the intermediate layer (vastus lateralis and vastus medialis), and the deep layer from the vastus intermedius. You can also identify these three layers on the transverse or short-axis plane. Deep to the quadriceps tendon, you can visualize the suprapatellar fat pad as well as the prefemoral fat pad.

If the knee is then hyperflexed, the femoral trochlea can be visualized on long-axis planes. This allows examination of the articular cartilage of the trochlea.

Moving caudally (distally), one can examine the patellar tendon in both long-axis and short-axis views. As you move from cranial (proximal) to caudal (distal) over the tendon, be sure to do both long-axis scans and short-axis slides across the tendon. After looking from the patella to the tibial tubercle in long axis, rotate the probe 90° and look at the same structure in short axis. Deep to the patellar tendon, you can visualize the deep infrapatellar bursa, as well as Hoffa's fat pad, which can be seen intra-articularly.

The advantage of ultrasound for diagnosis of quadriceps tendon rupture was highlighted by LaRocco et al. [1] and Secko et al. [2]. Vreju et al. [3] used ultrasound to show changes at the distal potion of the patellar tendon and at the distal tuberosity in an athlete with Osgood-Schlatter's disease (Table 12.1).

## Medial Knee

The patient remains in the supine position with the knee still flexed, but the patient is asked to externally rotate the knee.

The examiner remains in the same position.

The transducer is oriented in a long-axis plane obliquely over the medial collateral ligament (MCL). One should examine the MCL from origin to insertion. To increase sensitivity of the exam, you can examine the MCL dynamically and have someone place the knee under valgus stress. You will also see the medial meniscus. As you track caudally, you should rotate the transducer forward to image the tendons of the pes complex. It is impossible to differentiate the three tendons (sartorius, gracilis, and semitendinosus). You

P.A. Smith, M.D.
Department of Orthopaedic Surgery, University of Missouri Hospitals and Clinics, Columbia, MO, USA

Columbia Orthopaedic Group, 1 South Keene Street, Columbia, MO 65201, USA
e-mail: psmithmudoc@aol.com

M.E. Thornburg, M.D. (✉)
Columbia Orthopaedic Group, 1 South Keene Street, Columbia, MO 65201, USA

University of Missouri, Columbia, MO, USA
e-mail: m.thornburg@columbiaorthogroup.com

J.M. Daniels and W.W. Dexter (eds.), *Basics of Musculoskeletal Ultrasound*,
DOI 10.1007/978-1-4614-3215-9_12, © Springer Science+Business Media New York 2013

**Table 12.1** Knee

| Patient position | Transducer position and description | Picture of scan and labeled structures | Pearls/pitfalls |
|---|---|---|---|
| *Anterior superior knee*<br>Patient in supine position, knee flexed 20–30°, with pillow under knee | Longitudinal or long-axis view<br>Probe superior to patella | Labeled structures<br>PAT—patella<br>QT—quadriceps tendon<br>SPR—suprapatellar recess<br>SPFP—suprapatellar fat pad | Start at the patella and scan both long- and short-axis views along the full length of the quad tendon. Try to visualize all three layers<br>A panoramic view allows visualization of the patella and the quad tendon insertion. Some call this the "wind blowing snow over the mountain" view. (The patella looks like the mountain, the intact quad like snow blowing off the peak) |
| | Transverse or short-axis view<br>Probe superior to patella 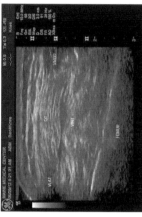 | Labeled structures<br>Femur<br>QT—quadriceps tendon<br>VMED—vastus medialis<br>VLAT—vastus lateralis<br>VINT—vastus intermedius | |

Dynamic and sono-palpation views are key when evaluating full-thickness tears. They can be difficult to diagnose

Once the suprapatellar space is identified, joint effusion is easily drained under MSK/US guidance

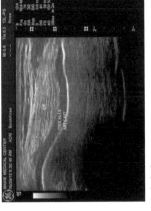

Short-axis view
Prcbe just above patella

Labeled structures
QT—quadriceps tendon
TROCHLEA
ART CART—articular cartilage

*Anterior superior knee*
Patient in supine position, maximum flexion

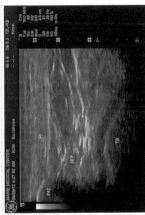

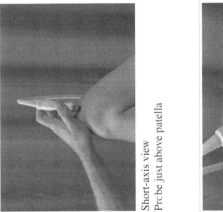

Long-axis view
Probe inferior to patella

Labeled structures
PAT—patella
PT—patellar tendon
TIB—tibia
HFP—Hoffman's fat pad

*Anterior inferior knee*
Patient in supine position, knee flexed 20–30°,
with pillow under knee

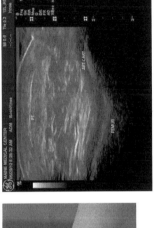

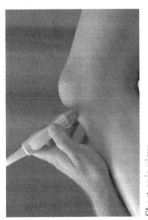

Short-axis view
Probe inferior to patella

Labeled structures
PT—patellar tendon
ART CART—articular cartilage
FEMUR

(continued)

**Table 12.1** (continued)

| Patient position | Transducer position and description | Picture of scan and labeled structures | Pearls/pitfalls |
|---|---|---|---|
| *Medial knee*<br>Patient is supine, with knee flexed 20–30°, with pillow under knee, knee slightly externally rotated | Long-axis view<br>Probe over medial joint line | Labeled structures<br>MCL—medial collateral ligament<br>MM—medial meniscus<br>TIBIA<br>FEMUR | Find the joint line. The MCL will be just below the skin. Have an assistant apply valgus stress. Observe MCL with full extension and 30° flexion. Observe all of tendons, including insertions<br>Also, try to find the medial retinaculum and dynamically look for subluxation, bony avulsions, and injury to MCL. Injuries at the femoral origin are associated with injury to the medial patellofemoral ligament<br>Find the pes anserine bursa Insertion of sartorius gracilis, semitendinosus |
| | Long-axis view—pes<br>Slide transducer distally over joint line 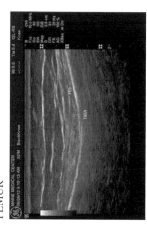 | Labeled structures<br>TIBIA<br>PES—pes anserine | |
| | Short-axis view—pes<br>As above 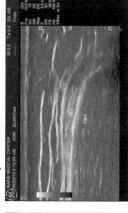 | Labeled structures<br>TIBIA<br>PES | |

*Lateral knee*
Patient supine, knee slightly internally rotated and flexed at 20–30°

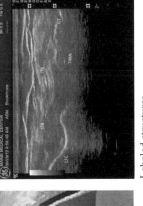

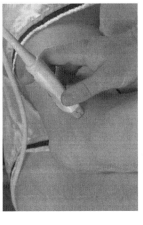

Long-axis view
Lateral joint line

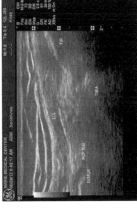

Labeled structures
ITB—iliotibial band
GT—Gerdy's tubercle
LFC—lateral femoral condyle
TIBIA

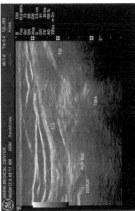

Long-axis view
Distal probe at fibular head, rotate proximal probe anteriorly to evaluate LCL

Labeled structures
POP TEN—popliteus tendon
LCL—lateral collateral ligament
FIB—fibular head
FEMUR
TIBIA

Identify Gerdy's tubercle and evaluate

- Iliotibial band
- Lateral meniscus

Evaluate for meniscal cysts: Have patient flex knee as much as possible and place transducer on the joint line to evaluate lateral meniscus cysts

Deep to the proximal portion of the IT band, the popliteus tendon can be evaluated

Injection through the IT band into the posterior space between the tendon and bone can be easily done in this position

When identifying a Baker's cyst, evaluate lateral to the medial head of the gastrocnemius at its origin. Other space-occupying lesions can be mistaken for Baker's cysts

When the patient is prone, the vessels may collapse. Having the patient flex and extend the knee allows the vessels to be seen

(continued)

**Table 12.1** (continued)

| Patient position | Transducer position and description | Picture of scan and labeled structures | Pearls/pitfalls |
|---|---|---|---|
| *Posterior knee*<br>Patient is in prone (face down) position, knee completely extended<br>May place a small pillow under tibia for patient comfort | <br>Long-axis view<br>Medial | <br>Labeled structures<br>SMT—semimembranosus tendon<br>MFC—medial femoral condyle | Start medially, and identify<br>Sartorius tendon<br>Saphenous nerve<br>Medial femoral condyle<br>Medial head of gastrocnemius<br>Semimembranosus<br>Semitendinosus<br>Then scan laterally to the popliteal fossa, popliteal artery, and popliteal vein (use Doppler setting)<br>Then scan to the lateral aspect of knee; see the peroneal nerve at fibular head and bicep femoris |
| | <br>Long-axis view<br>Lateral | <br>Labeled structures<br>FH—fibular head<br>BT—biceps femoris tendon | |
| | <br>Short-axis view<br>Medial | <br>Labeled structures<br>MFC—medial femoral condyle<br>SMT—semimembranosus tendon<br>STT—semitendinosus tendon<br>SN—sural nerve<br>MHG—medial head gastrocnemius muscle | |

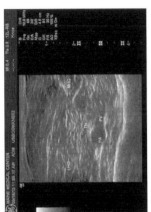

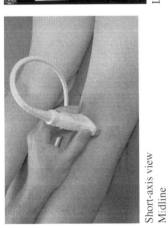

Short-axis view
Midline

Labeled structures
MHG—medial head of gastrocnemius
LHG—lateral head of gastrocnemius
TN—tibial nerve
PA—popliteal artery
PV—popliteal vein

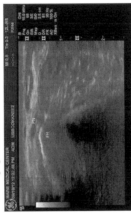

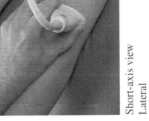

Short-axis view
Lateral

Labeled structures
FH—fibular head
PN—peroneal nerve

may see fluid over the pes that may be indicative of pes anserine bursitis.

Ultrasound evaluation of the pes bursa has been shown to be very helpful, both diagnostically and therapeutically. Yoon et al. [4] found value in the use of ultrasonography in patients with pes anserine bursitis as an adjunct to further therapy, such as a local corticosteroid injection.

Injury to the medial retinaculum and attachment of the medial patellofemoral ligament may be evident following a patellar dislocation injury. In fact, Trikha et al. [5] performed a promising study comparing preoperative ultrasound to operative findings in ten patients following acute patellar dislocation. They found a strong correlation with medial retinacular injury, particularly with bony avulsions on ultrasound, to the surgical findings, and also found that fluid on ultrasound around the MCL origin correlated with injury to the medial patellofemoral ligament (MPFL).

Park et al. [6] found ultrasound correlated with MRI in 86 % of cases for meniscus tears and correlated with MRI in 85 % of the cases with no meniscus tear. Overall, the positive predictive value for a tear was 76 %, and the negative predictive value was 92 %. Also, Wareluk and Szopinski [7] in 2011 showed similar findings comparing ultrasound diagnosis of meniscus tear to arthroscopic evaluation with a sensitivity rating of 85 % and a specificity of 86 % for ultrasound. Nevertheless, MRI is still the gold standard for the most accurate delineation of meniscus tear.

## Lateral Knee

The patient remains in the supine position with the knee flexed and is asked to internally rotate the knee.

The examiner remains in the same position.

The iliotibial (IT) band is evaluated in long axis starting superiorly and tracking down to Gerdy's tubercle. You should identify the joint line and lateral meniscus. If a meniscal cyst is present, you may forcefully flex the knee to try and produce bulging of the cyst. In fact, Smillie [8] and Reagan et al. [9] showed that between 84 and 86 % of cystic menisci had associated lateral meniscus tears. These meniscal cysts may be seen nicely on ultrasound, particularly to facilitate aspiration or a steroid injection. Rutten et al. [10] and Sorrentino et al. [11] compared ultrasound to MRI for evaluation of meniscal cysts and found a sensitivity of 94 % and specificity of 100 % for ultrasound.

To examine the lateral collateral ligament (LCL), extend the knee and place the transducer on the femoral head. Rotate the transducer anteriorly until the LCL appears in the image. It can be difficult to assess the true status of the LCL, and you may consider an MRI to better assess all ligamentous structures. Deep to the proximal portion of the LCL, you can see the popliteal tendon in its bony groove.

## Posterior Knee

The patient is placed in a prone (lying face down) position with the knee in a fully extended position. In some cases, you may have the patient flex the knee slightly to obtain a more dynamic scan, especially when looking for a Baker's cyst and its communication with the joint. For ease of the exam, the examiner may keep the same position and reach over to the opposite side of the table to examine the posterior structures. It may be necessary to stand or sit on the edge of the exam table for quality and comfort. The ultrasound machine remains on the far side of the table.

As you begin to scan posteriorly, start medially in a short-axis plane; you should identify the sartorius (muscle fibers), gracilis tendon, and the semitendinosus tendon located behind the semimembranosus tendon.

In the popliteal fossa, you can identify the popliteal artery, popliteal vein, and tibial nerve (going deep to superficial). In the long axis, you can identify the posterior cruciate ligament. In between the semimembranosus tendon medially and the medial head of the gastrocnemius laterally may be a space-occupying mass with a wide spectrum of appearances. Typically, you can see the base located along the semimembranosus tendon, the tendon of the medial head of the gastrocnemius, and the posterior capsule. The base of the cyst is often smaller than the superficial portion. A small stalk connecting the base with the posterior joint is not always seen. When making the diagnosis of Baker's cyst using ultrasound and physical exam criteria, it is important to locate the cyst just lateral to medial gastrocnemius muscle; otherwise, other pathology (masses) cannot be completely ruled out.

As you move to the posterolateral aspect of the knee, you can examine the posterolateral corner and biceps femoris. You may examine the biceps femoris muscle and tendon in both long- and short-axis planes. It is often helpful to find the myotendinous junction of the two heads of the biceps femoris, as this is a common injury in sports. From here you can follow it to its insertion at the fibular head. Here you can also visualize the lateral femoral condyle, the lateral meniscus, and the lateral tibial plateau.

## Probe Selection/Settings

Transducer should have a 5–10-MHz linear array. If your machine has presets, use them. Otherwise, set for shallow depth.

## Ultrasound as a Diagnostic Tool for the Knee

Joint synovitis can be appreciated by using the color Doppler setting to search for neovascularization. Ultrasound can also help diagnose subtle joint effusions correlating with acute flares in osteoarthritis patients in the absence of other obvious clinical findings.

A recent systematic review confirms that accuracy is better with the use of ultrasound-guided intra-articular injection and that short-term outcomes are improved, but there is no appreciable difference in long-term outcomes compared to standard injection based on palpating anatomic landmarks [12]. A study from the *British Journal of Nursing* on ultrasound-guided intra-articular knee injections or aspirations supports the concept that incorporating musculoskeletal ultrasound into clinical practice leads to significant improvements in patient care. This study also commented on the appreciation patients had for ultrasound-guided procedures [13].

Ultrasound can be utilized to precisely inject anesthetic into a tendon sheath and evaluate the patient's response. Patients localize their symptoms, and ultrasound can then be used to safely deliver medication to affected tissue with precision, and then clinical response is monitored. Tendon sonography and injections of tendon sheaths can be challenging but ultrasound has the advantage of potentially reducing risk of iatrogenic tendon injury by allowing for increased accuracy.

## Red Flags

When evaluating the knee, many conditions will need to be confirmed with MRI or other modality. One should recognize the limitations of ultrasound at the present time. It can be very helpful and even diagnostic in patellar tendon and quadriceps tendon ruptures. If these are suspected, it requires early referral for surgical consideration.

It can also be useful in differentiating a cellulitic process from a true abscess (i.e., fluid formation.[1]). If one can identify a cystic type structure, it may be helpful to aspirate under ultrasound guidance.

## Pearls and Pitfalls

At this point in time, there is a limited role for ultrasound in the knee. The most useful role is in the assessment of tendon lesions. It is particularly helpful in quadriceps and patellar tendon injuries/ruptures. It is as or more effective than MRI for evaluating chronic tendonosis. It can also be helpful in ultrasound-guided injections in these settings: Baker's cyst, fluid aspiration, tendinitis conditions, and so forth.

Ultrasound allows for dynamic examinations, and you can easily compare to the contralateral side. One study showed a reliable positive predictive value (100 %) of injury to the posterolateral corner with a positive dynamic ultrasound stress test (>10.5 mm).

As we advance our ultrasound capabilities, ultrasound will play a larger role in the diagnosis of injuries or pathologies of the knee. It is certainly gaining ground in diagnosing meniscal pathology, and in cases where MRI is not advisable, it may be the next best modality.

## Clinical Experience

1. Obtain a panoramic view of the quadriceps tendon and its insertion into the patellar for the "wind blowing snow off the peak of the mountain" view. Attempt to demonstrate all levels (three) of the quad tendon.
2. Obtain a view of the patella and trochlea with the knee in complete flexion.
3. Identify and scan area of the knee where therapeutic injections can be used.
   (a) Suprapatellar space.
   (b) Space between IT band and bone on lateral aspect of knee.
4. With the help of an assistant, demonstrate dynamic testing of the MCL with the knee in full extension and 30° of flexion.

## References

1. LaRocco BG, Zlupko G, Sierzenski P. Ultrasound diagnosis of quadriceps tendon rupture. J Emerg Med. 2008;35(3):293–5.
2. Secko M, Diaz M, Paladino L. Ultrasound diagnosis of quadriceps tendon tear in an uncooperative patient. J Emerg Trauma Shock. 2011;4(4):521–2.
3. Vreju F, Ciurea P, Rosu A. Osgood-Schlatter disease—ultrasonic diagnostic. Med Ultrason. 2010;12(4):336–9.
4. Yoon HS, Kim SE, Suh YR, Seo YI, Kim HA. Correlation between ultrasonographic findings and the response to corticosteroid injection in pes anserinus tendinobursitis syndrome in knee osteoarthritis patients. J Korean Med Sci. 2005;20(1):109–12.
5. Trikha SP, Acton D, O'Reilly M, Curtis MJ, Bell J. Acute lateral dislocation of the patella: correlation of ultrasound scanning with operative findings. Injury. 2003;34(8):568–71.
6. Park GY, Kim JM, Lee SM, Lee MY. The value of ultrasonography in the detection of meniscal tears diagnosed by magnetic resonance imaging. Am J Phys Med Rehabil. 2008;87(1):14–20.
7. Wareluk P, Szopinski KT. Value of modern sonography in the assessment of meniscal lesions. Eur J Radiol. 2012;81(9):2366–9.
8. Smillie IS. Injuries of the knee joint. 5th ed. London: Churchill-Livingstone; 1978. p. 94–8.
9. Reagan WD, McConkey JP, Loomer RL, Davidson RG. Cysts of the lateral meniscus: arthroscopy vs arthroscopy plus open cystectomy. Arthroscopy. 1989;5:274–81.
10. Rutten M, Collins JM, van Kampen A, Jager GJ. Meniscal cysts: detection with high-resolution sonography. AJR. 1998;171:491–6.
11. Sorrentino F, Iovane A, Nicosia A, Vaccari A, Candela F, Cimino PG, et al. High resolution ultrasonography (HRUS) of the meniscal cyst of the knee: our experience. Radiol Med. 2007;112(5):732–9.
12. Gilliland CA, Salazar LD, Borchers JR. Ultrasound versus ultrasonic guidance for intra-articular and peri-articular injection: a systematic review. Phys Sportsmed. 2012;39(3):121–31.
13. El Miedany Y. Musculoskeletal US: examining the joints. Br J Nurs. 2012;21(6):340–4.

---

[1] An infectious effusion cannot be differentiated from an infiltrating one on musculoskeletal ultrasound. Aspiration is required to make a definitive diagnosis.

# Hip

# 13

## John Charles Hill and Matthew S. Leiszler

## Probe Selections and Presets

A linear transducer at 10–13 MHz will allow the best visualization for thin patients, especially for the lateral hip structures. A curvilinear 5-MHz probe is often necessary for muscular or obese patients to allow adequate penetration and visualization of the joint and deeper hip structures. Generally, it is best to start with a high-frequency linear transducer and then switch to a curvilinear transducer if unable to visualize adequately. Use the highest frequency transducer that provides adequate penetration. If your machine has hip presets, start with those. If the hip joint is deeper than 6 cm, then a 5-MHz curvilinear transducer set at 10–12 cm of depth with two focal zones will give the best visualization.

## Approach to the Joint

### Anterior Hip

The patient should be supine on the examination table, leg relaxed, and with minimal flexion of hip. The hip should be slightly externally rotated and the knee slightly flexed. Examiner is seated on an adjustable rolling stool, sitting by the side of an adjustable table next to the hip that is being examined. The ultrasound screen should be toward the head of the patient or across the table for easiest viewing (Table 13.1).

Place the transducer in a longitudinal (sagittal) plane, long-axis view, near the inguinal ligament. Slide the transducer laterally and medially to identify the hip joint and femoral vessels.

Then turn the transducer 90° to a transverse or short-axis (horizontal) position to confirm the center of the hip joint and observe that the femoral vessels are to the right of the visual field.

The acetabulum can then be identified as a thin cusp to the left of the femoral head; the labrum is attached to it and appears as a triangular and mixed echogenic structure. The femoral head flattens to form the femoral neck, and overlying this is the joint capsule.

If osteoarthritis is present, there may be an irregular appearance of the femoral head, narrowing of the joint space, and osteophyte formation on the acetabulum.

Synovitis may appear as a thickened hypoechoic structure within the joint space (average thickness is 5.2 mm; pathologic thickness >8–9 mm) and may be mistaken as a large joint effusion. Turn on the Doppler setting and note the amount of vascularity present. A large amount of vascularity is indicative of synovitis, as opposed to the absence of vessels in an effusion. Both may be present.

"Femoral acetabulum impingement" is a term used to describe some factors that may be associated with premature arthritis of the hip. While best identified using radiographs, musculoskeletal ultrasound may be useful in identifying incongruence of the femoral head and the acetabulum. While most patients have a combination, there are two distinct types of impingement: cam (the femoral neck is too thick or the "ball is too big for the socket") and pincer (the acetabulum is too large or the "socket is too big for the ball").

The cam-shaped (thickened) femoral neck is less distinct and almost blends in with femoral head. The joint capsule closely adheres to the femoral neck. The acetabulum is distinct and pointed in appearance. The labrum is frequently blunted and detached from the acetabulum. These patients may require both diagnostic and therapeutic injection if it is unclear whether impingement is the pain generator.

The entire labrum cannot be seen with ultrasound, but the anterior superior labrum is easily visualized. Start by scanning the anterior hip joint in both long- and short-axis planes. The normal labrum is triangular, slightly echogenic, and is firmly attached to the acetabulum. An acute disruption of the labrum is evidenced by a rounded or blunted

J.C. Hill, D.O. (✉) • M.S. Leiszler, M.D.
Family Medicine and Sports Medicine, University of Colorado School of Medicine, 2000 South Colorado Boulevard, Tower 1, Suite 4500, Denver, CO 80222, USA
e-mail: John.Hill@ucdenver.edu

**Table 13.1** Hip

| Patient position | Transducer position and description | Picture of scan and labeled structures | Pearls/pitfalls |
|---|---|---|---|
| *Anterior hip*<br><br>Patient should be supine on the examination table, leg relaxed, and with no flexion of hip. The hip should be slightly externally rotated and knee slightly flexed. Examiner is seated on an adjustable, rolling stool, by the side of an adjustable table next to the hip that is being examined. Ultrasound screen should be toward the head of the patient or across the table for easiest viewing | Lean patients: 10–13-MHz linear probe<br><br>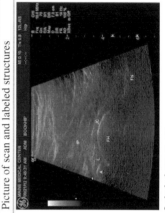<br><br>Longitudinal or long axis, over anterior hip<br>Obese, muscular patients and deep structures: 5-MHz curved probe | 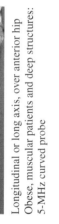<br><br>Labeled structures<br>IP—iliopsoas<br>FH—femoral head<br>FN—femoral neck<br>A—acetabulum<br>L—labrum<br>JC—joint capsule | Evaluate<br>• Femoral acetabular joint<br>• Joint capsule (average width 5 mm; >8 mm = synovitis)<br>• Labrum—anterior portion can be visualized<br>• Iliopsoas tendon and bursa<br>Psoas bursa, if effusion is present, will be superficial to the capsule. The presence of effusion should be confirmed in both short and long axis<br>For hip joint injection, the examiner usually can inject into the capsule overlying the femoral neck if effusion is present<br>If injecting from superior approach, choosing an approach in which the femoral head is more convex will make approach to the capsule more difficult<br>Using a 10-cm, 22-gauge spinal needle allows for adequate depth penetration to hip joint for most injections |
| *Lateral hip*<br><br>Patient should be in decubitus position on the examination table, hips slightly flexed to help with stability, and a pillow placed between the two knees to reduce discomfort. Examiner is seated on an adjustable, rolling stool, by the side of an adjustable table next to the hip that is being examined. Ultrasound screen should be toward the head of the patient or across the table for easiest viewing | Transducer: start with 10–13-MHz linear transducer. For deeper structures, switch to 5-MHz curved transducer<br><br>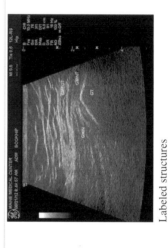<br><br>Long axis, over greater trochanter/gluteal tendons | 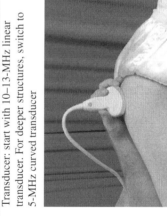<br><br>Labeled structures<br>GT—greater trochanter<br>GMIN—gluteus minimus muscle<br>GMINT—gluteus minimus tendon<br>GMEDT—gluteus medius tendon | Evaluate<br>• Greater trochanteric bursa (usually <2 mm, >5 mm = effusion)<br>• Gluteus medius and gluteus medius bursa muscle deep to IT band, bursa deep to muscle; usually a potential space, if present, may indicate inflammation<br>When inflamed, piriformis muscle insertion tendon is usually indistinguishable from the gluteus medius because it becomes hypoechoic (dark)<br>Visualizing the contralateral side is useful to confirm abnormal findings on affected side<br>Is trochanteric bursitis the source of pain?<br>Lateral hip pain can come from the gluteus medius bursa, the gluteus maximus (trochanteric) bursa, or insertional tendon pathology<br>If you see fluid in the trochanteric bursa, do not assume that is the only area of inflammation. Frequently, the gluteus medius bursa will need to be injected at the same time |

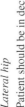

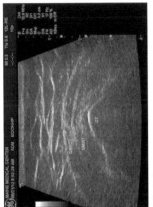

Transverse or short axis, over greater trochanter/
gluteal tendons

Labeled structures
GT—greater trochanter
GMINT—gluteus minimus tendon
GMEDT—gluteus medius tendon

appearance and a thin hypoechoic space between the acetabulum and the labrum.

The iliopsoas tendon and bursa can also be easily visualized with musculoskeletal ultrasound. Start with the transducer in a longitudinal or long-axis (sagittal) plane near the inguinal ligament. Slide the transducer laterally and medially to identify the hip joint and the iliopsoas tendon just superficial to the joint. Then turn the transducer to a transverse or short-axis position to confirm the center of the hip joint; note the round appearance of the psoas major muscle situated here.

The iliopsoas tendon lies directly above the hip joint and normally has a gray, mixed echogenic appearance similar to the rectus femoris muscle, which is directly above it. The psoas bursa is normally not seen unless it is distended because of inflammation or infection. When it is present, it is a thin, anechoic black space directly above the hip joint and below the iliopsoas tendon.

## Lateral Hip

The patient should be in decubitus position on the examination table, hips slightly flexed to help with stability, and a pillow placed between the two knees to reduce discomfort. The examiner is seated in an adjustable rolling stool, sitting by the side of an adjustable table next to the hip that is being examined. The ultrasound screen should be toward the head of the patient or across the table for easiest viewing.

Start scanning with the transducer in a longitudinal (coronal) plane near the widest part of the hip. Slide the transducer anteriorly and posteriorly and angle the beam to identify the greater trochanter. Turn the transducer to a short-axis position to confirm the center of the trochanter, and then slide the transducer superiorly and inferiorly to identify the top of the lateral femur. With the transducer in a long-axis plane near the posterosuperior aspect of the lateral femur, the margin between the trochanter and the less hyperechoic iliotibial band is the trochanteric bursa or the subcutaneous bursa of the gluteus maximus. Normally, the trochanteric bursa is a potential space and measures less than 2 mm. When inflamed, it is common to see effusions greater than 5–10 mm.

Next, identify the gluteus medius insertion and gluteus medius bursa. Start with the transducer in a longitudinal (coronal) plane near the widest part of the hip. Slide the transducer anteriorly and posteriorly and angle the beam to identify the superior greater trochanter. Turn the transducer to a short-axis position to confirm the center of the trochanter, and then slide the transducer superiorly and inferiorly to identify the insertion of the gluteus medius tendon on the lateral femur.

The gluteus medius tendon is echoic in appearance and is deep to the iliotibial (IT) band, inserting on the anterosuperior portion of the proximal femur. The bursa is normally not seen because it is a potential space, but when inflamed it is anechoic in appearance, just deep to the gluteus medius tendon and anterior to the trochanteric bursa.

To identify the piriformis muscle insertion, start with the transducer in a longitudinal or long-axis (coronal) plane near the posterior proximal femur. Slide the transducer anteriorly and posteriorly and angle the beam to identify the posterosuperior femur. Then turn the transducer to a short-axis position to identify the fibers of the piriformis tendon as it inserts on the posterosuperior femur, deep to the gluteus maximus muscle and parallel to the gluteus medius tendon. The normal appearance of this tendon is slightly echogenic and appears almost indistinguishable from the gluteus medius tendon. When inflamed, it is densely hypoechoic near the insertion and the remainder of the muscle is mildly hypoechoic. The sciatic nerve is located deep to this muscle near the origin.

## Common Problems

### Are Blood Vessels in the Path of My Needle?

First, visualize femoral vessels in both short- and long-axis views. Use color flow Doppler to ensure that femoral artery and vein are medial to your injection path. Next, identify the lateral femoral circumflex artery as it crosses the joint capsule in various locations. In a long-axis view, use color flow Doppler to identify the location when mapping the potential path your needle will take to the joint capsule or to the iliopsoas bursa.

Lastly, determine if an inferior or superior approach is preferable to avoid vessels. The superior approach is used when the needle is entering the skin above the transducer and approaches the bursa and joint capsule obliquely. The inferior approach is used when the needle enters below the transducer and approaches the bursa and joint capsule perpendicularly. This is generally the easiest approach, but it is the one most likely to encounter the lateral femoral circumflex artery.

### Is Impingement or Labrum the Pain Generator?

An injection into the femoral acetabulum joint space can be both diagnostic and therapeutic if you are unclear whether impingement or a small labral tear is the pain generator. The iliopsoas tendon can also be the source of significant hip pain. Initially, if the patient is pain-free after a joint injection, the cause of the pain is from within the joint (osteoarthritis, impingement/labrum). If the patient's pain returns in an hour or two, then the likely cause of pain is the iliopsoas tendon and not from the joint. The psoas tendon can then be injected with lidocaine. The cessation of pain confirms the diagnosis.

## Is Trochanteric Bursitis the Source of Pain?

Lateral hip pain can come from the gluteus medius bursa, the gluteus maximus (trochanteric) bursa, or an insertional tendon tear or tendinopathy. If you see fluid in the trochanteric bursa, do not assume that it is the only area of inflammation. Frequently, the gluteus medius bursa will need to be injected at the same time.

## Where Is the Pain from Piriformis Syndrome?

The pain is most commonly felt along the sciatic nerve, but the more common site of injury is near the insertion at the lateral femur. If the piriformis tendon is hypoechoic and stands out from the other tendons inserting on the greater trochanter, then this is likely where the injury is located and the treatment should be focused here.

## Red Flags

If there are concerns for infection of the hip (i.e., warmth of the joint, fever, acute onset), ultrasound is unable to differentiate infection vs. effusion of the hip joint. However, a sample of the joint fluid can be obtained for analysis to assist in obtaining the diagnosis.

An injection should not be attempted if there is any possibility of vascular structures in the planned pathway to the joint.

## Pearls and Pitfalls

### Pearls

- Visualize the contralateral joint to confirm abnormal findings on affected side.
- The rectus femoris lies superficial to the psoas. The psoas lies superficial to the capsule.

- Psoas bursa, if effusion is present, will be superficial to the capsule. The presence of effusion should be confirmed in both short and long axis.
- For hip joint injection, the examiner usually can inject into the capsule overlying the femoral neck, if effusion is present.
- Using a 100-cm, 22-gauge spinal needle allows for adequate depth penetration to the hip joint for most injections.

### Pitfall

- If injecting from a superior approach, choosing an approach in which the femoral head is more convex will make approach to the capsule more difficult.

## Clinical Exercise/Homework

1. Record a picture of the anterior view of the hip joint. Identify the anterior labrum, iliopsoas tendon, and the femoral and circumflex vessels. Please use Doppler setting to identify the vessels.
2. Record a picture of the lateral view of the hip. Identify the potential space of the greater trochanteric bursa and the insertion of the gluteus medius and the piriformis tendons.

## Suggested Reading

Bianchi S, Martinoli C. Ultrasound of the musculoskeletal system. New York, NY: Springer; 2007.

European Society of Musculoskeletal Radiology. "European Society of Musculoskeletal Radiology Guidelines." *Essr.org*. ESSR European Society of Musculoskeletal Radiology. n.d. Web. October 2012.

Jacobson JA. Fundamentals of musculoskeletal ultrasound. Philadelphia, PA: Saunders Elsevier; 2007.

McNally E. Practical musculoskeletal ultrasound. Philadelphia, PA: Elsevier; 2007.

Stoller DW. Stoller's atlas of orthopaedics and sports medicine. Baltimore, MD: Lippincott Williams & Wilkins; 2008.

# Groin

Anthony E. Joseph

## Approach to the Patient

Patients with groin pain should first be evaluated for hip pathology. This is described in a separate chapter. The evaluation techniques described in this chapter will require the patient to perform a number of dynamic maneuvers while the probe is placed on various areas of the patient's groin. A professional, yet comforting, environment and respect for the patient's privacy are necessary to obtain optimal scans.

## Evaluation of the Musculature of the Groin

The patient should be interviewed fully clothed first, then asked to change into a gown, shorts, and/or sheets. The procedure should be described to the patient, and an assistant should be present at all times during the examination.

The patient is placed in a supine (lying, face up) position and asked to relax "their hips" to allow both hips to abduct while flexing their knees. This allows easy access to the first landmark used: the pubic symphysis. A transverse or short-axis view is obtained and evaluated for bony irregularity, asymmetry, and presence of fluid. These findings can often be seen in the asymptomatic population, but if sono-palpation (examiner applies gentle pressure to the area being scanned with the probe) reproduces the patient's pain, they are significant. The patient is then asked to straighten their legs and perform alternating leg lifts to see if this reproduces their pain and/or shows movement at the symphysis. At this time, move the probe superiorly, then to the right and to the left, so the superior pubic ramus and pubic tubercle can be evaluated. This is a common site for tendinopathies associated with sports-related groin pain.

A.E. Joseph, M.D. (✉)
Portneuf Medical Center, Pocatello Orthopaedic and Sports Medicine Institute/Idaho State University, 333 North 18th Avenue, Pocatello, ID 83201, USA
e-mail: joseanth@isu.edu

The probe is moved laterally toward the hip joint (perform on both sides) over the pubic tubercle to evaluate the adductor tendon insertion attachment of the musculature of the hip. These structures are evaluated for tears and/or signs of tendinopathy. The rectus abdominis muscle is first viewed as the probe moves superiorly as they connect over the pubis bone. Rotate the probe 90° to also obtain long-axis views of these tendons. The adductor tendons next come into view as the probe is moved laterally. There are three layers from the most superficial to the deepest: the adductor longus, adductor brevis, and adductor magnus. As the probe moves medially, the gracilis muscle can also be evaluated.

Next, evaluate the ASIS (anterior superior iliac spine) and the origin of the tensor fascia latae and sartorius muscle along with the AIIS (anterior inferior iliac spine) origin of the rectus femoris muscle. This is especially important when evaluating adolescents, because these locations are common areas of injury in this group. Reproduction of pain by sono-palpation helps confirm that these tendons are pain generators (ASIS—hip abduction, knee flexion, hold knee down, and have patient forcefully adduct hip. AIIS—resist leg lift) (Table 14.1).

## Common Problems

### Snapping Hip Syndrome

Patients may present with the complaint of a painful "snapping" of the hip. Rarely, this can be as a result of acetabulum impingement or labral pathology. More commonly it occurs because the iliopsoas tendon is "snapping" against the anterior aspect of the hip joint, ilium, or ilioperitoneal eminence (Table 14.2).

This can be evaluated by having an assistant internally and externally rotate the foot with the patient in both full hip extension and then at 45° flexion. The probe is placed over the anterior position of the in short axis, and the AIIS to see if this maneuver reproduces the patient's symptoms and to observe any tendon displacement.

**Table 14.1** Evaluation of superficial musculature of hip and groin

| Patient position | Transducer position and description | Picture of scan and labeled structures | Pearls/pitfalls |
|---|---|---|---|
| Patient supine (face up) and extends knees | Transducer = 7.5- to 13-MHz linear array 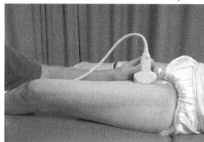 <br> Longitudinal or long-axis view <br> The probe is placed long axis, on the iliac crest | 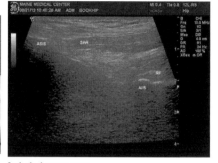 <br> Labeled structures <br> ASIS—anterior superior iliac spine <br> AIIS—anterior inferior iliac spine <br> RF—rectus femoris <br> SAR—sartorius | Palpation of iliac crest and anterior aspect allows for identification of ASIS and AIIS <br> Evaluate the superficial musculature of hip and groin |

Another common location where snapping hip syndrome occurs is where the anterior portion of the iliotibial tract subluxes over the greater trochanter of the femur. This can be evaluated by placement of the probe over the greater trochanter while having the patient lie on his/her side with the affected hip facing upward. Ask the patient to then flex, extend, and rotate the hip to reproduce the symptoms. Reproduction of the symptoms with sono-palpation or observation that the IT band snapping reproduces the symptoms makes the diagnosis.

## Evaluation of Hernias

Patients presenting with groin pain may not have a musculoskeletal problem but a tear or weakness in the fascia around the lower abdomen and groin. Patients may be frustrated because this groin pathology is sometimes difficult to localize; patients with hernias may present to orthopedic surgeons, while patients with musculoskeletal problems may present to general surgeons. If the patient has two or more conditions (a fairly common occurrence) and only one is diagnosed and treated, the symptoms may persist (Table 14.3).

As a clinical sonographer's experience grows and scanning skills improve, so will the capacity to help these patients. For this reason, we have included the following discussion about hernias in this musculoskeletal ultrasound chapter.

The patient should be evaluated in a supine (lying face up) position, knee slightly flexed, and hip slightly externally rotated. Place the probe in a short axis position over the anterior hip joint. Slide the probe medially and laterally until the femoral artery and vein are seen. The use of color Doppler may not be needed. The femoral nerve is located just laterally to these vessels. (The mnemonic NAVEL is useful to remember—nerve, artery, vein, empty, lymphatics.) Ask the patient to perform a Valsalva maneuver. Observe the area medial to the femoral vein (to the "empty" space in NAVEL) for a bulging of a femoral hernia. During this type of scanning, the patient is required to perform the Valsalva maneuver quite often and for a prolonged period of time. An easy way to perform the maneuver is to have the patient place the back of his/her hand up against the mouth and to blow out against the hand. The patient is easily able to hold a long Valsalva with varying pressure in this fashion.

The next area evaluated is medial and superior to the femoral triangle. It is key to be able to identify the epigastric vessels. Their position allows one to differentiate a direct hernia (below the vessels) from an indirect hernia (above the vessels). Take the probe and move it superiorly and medially until the border of the rectus abdominis muscle is found. Turn on the color Doppler and scan for the inferior epigastric artery and vein. The probe is then canted between longitudinal or long-axis and transverse or short-axis positions then moved laterally and inferiorly to find its origin at the iliac artery and vein. They will appear at the level of the inguinal ligament. An alternate method would be to place one gloved finger in the inguinal canal just as one checks for an indirect hernia clinically. The finger goes into the external ring. The probe in the other hand can then follow the canal up to the internal ring. The cord to the testicle can be identified, and the inferior epigastric vessels can be identified. Again, have the patient perform an extended Valsalva maneuver and identify any bulges.

## Sports Hernia

This entity has been described in the literature and given a number of different names over the years. It may have been

**Table 14.2** Evaluation of patient for snapping hip syndrome

| Patient position | Transducer position and description | Picture of scan and labeled structures | Pearls/pitfalls |
|---|---|---|---|
| Patient supine. Scan in this position, then ask patient to flex hip 45–90° as much as tolerated and rescan | 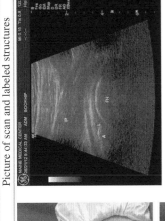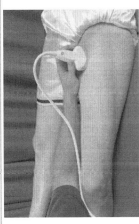Long-axis view<br>The probe is placed over the hip joint | 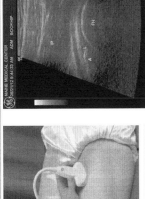Labeled structures<br>IP—iliopsoas<br>A—acetabulum<br>L—labrum<br>FH—femoral head | In adolescents, sono-palpation of these areas may reproduce pain if patient has apophysitis<br>Have assistant take foot and internally and externally rotate. Observe for snapping. Do this in flexion, then repeat procedure over ASIS<br>Snapping hip syndrome can rarely be caused by labral pathology or femoral acetabulum impingement. In the majority of cases, it is caused either by the iliopsoas or IT band snapping over a structure<br>*Also*<br>To assess the sartorius muscle (attaches to ASIS):<br>Have patient flex knee, abduct hip. Have patient forcefully adduct against resistance<br>To assess the rectus femoris (attaches to AIIS), have patient resist leg lift |
| Patient on non-affected side, affected hip side up. The patient is then asked to flex, extend, or rotate the hip to reproduce symptoms | 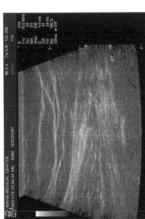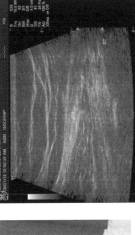Long-axis view<br>Probe placed over greater trochanter of femur | 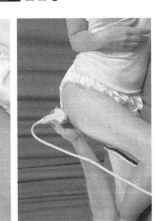Labeled structures<br>ITB—iliotibial band<br>GT—greater trochanter | The "snapping" should be observed to make the diagnosis |

**Table 14.3** Evaluation of the pubic symphysis

| Patient position | Transducer position and description | Picture of scan and labeled structures | Pearls/pitfalls |
|---|---|---|---|
| The patient is supine (face up). Have patient flex knees about 45–60°, then abduct hips | 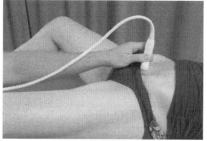<br>Transverse or short-axis view<br>Probe is placed on pubic symphysis in transverse position (horizontal or short-axis view) | 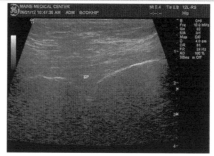<br>Labeled structures<br>SP—symphysis pubis | Evaluate the patient when fully clothed at first. Explain the procedure, then have the patient change into shorts, gown. Use sheets to ensure patient privacy and comfort<br>Always have an assistant present to help with the scan<br>Evaluate the pubic symphysis for bone irregularity and effusion<br>Evaluate for tears and tendinopathy<br>Have patient straighten knees and do alternate leg lifts; evaluate for movement and pain<br>Sono-palpation assists in determining if each structure is the pain generator |
| | 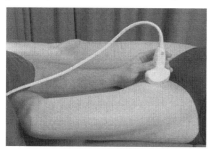<br>Long-axis view<br>Slide probe laterally over pubic ramus long axis to adductors | 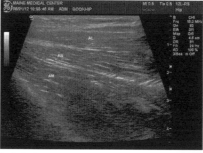<br>Labeled structures<br>AL—adductor longus<br>AB—adductor brevis<br>AM—adductor magnus | |
| | | 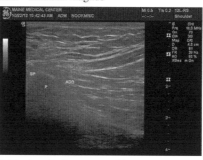<br>Adductor attachment to pubic ramus<br>Labeled structures<br>  ADD—adductor(s) tendon<br>  P—pubis<br>  SP—symphysis pubis | |

a "waste basket" diagnosis given when physicians were unable to find the cause of the patient's groin pain. We define this not as a "true hernia" but as a weakness or diastasis of the transversalis fascia that occurs at the rectus abdominis border or close to the external ring of the canal in the direct hernia region. This weakness is often not seen without an active Valsalva maneuver, so it has been difficult to image in the past. When the patient produces a prolonged Valsalva, the rectus abdominis may move medially or the cord may move laterally. Occasionally, the bladder may be seen moving into this defect. Ultrasound is the ideal modality to diagnose this problem, which is usually only symptomatic when the patient engages in strenuous activity producing increased abdominal pressure.

## The Postoperative Hip

Patient complaints of postoperative hip pain can be divided into main categories:

1. Pain over the front of the hip as a result of the snapping of the iliopsoas tendon over the anterior joint

2. Pain inside the joint from wear, loosening, or infection of the prosthesis

3. Pain laterally, related to tendinosis or tears of the gluteus musculature

If the patient has a complaint of pain over the anterior portion of the hip, the iliopsoas and its relationship to the acetabular component should be evaluated. As the prosthesis moves anteriorly during hip flexion, it will occasionally create friction between the prosthesis (especially if it is oversized) and the tendon. In both short- and long-axis views, irregularity and fibrosis of the iliopsoas muscle can be observed. Dynamic testing, such as having the patient flex and extend or internally or externally rotate the hip, accentuates this.

The joint should be evaluated for both excessive synovitis and effusion (a small amount of either is normal). Doppler settings help differentiate between the two. The Doppler will show increased vascularity of the area being scanned in patients with synovitis. If infection is suspected, aspiration of the effusion is necessary.

Postoperative pain in the posterior hip may also be related to partial or complete tears of the gluteus medius. The sciatic nerve may also be irritated from being stretched (axonotmesis, neurotmesis). This can be demonstrated by following the course of the sciatic nerve distally from its emergence below the piriformis muscle.

## Clinical Experience

1. Perform a dynamic scan of the pubic symphysis by having the patient alternate leg lifts. Identify the origin of the hernias adductors. Use dynamic methods that increase abdominal pressure to look for hernias.

2. Identify, scan, and record the ASIS, the origin of the sartorius, AIIS, and the origin of the rectus femoris muscle.

3. Identify, scan, and record the iliopsoas muscle as it passes over the anterior aspect of the hip joint by having the patient flex and extend the hip; then, with the help of an assistant, internally and externally rotate the foot while scanning the iliopsoas. In both positions, observe for snapping and impingement. Scan the lateral hip for movement of the anterior aspect of the IT band over the greater trochanter.

## Suggested Reading

Orchard JW, Read JW, Neophyton J, Garlick D. Groin pain associated with ultrasound finding of inguinal canal posterior wall deficiency in Australian Rules footballers. Br J Sports Med. 1998;32(2): 134–9.

Swan KG, Wolcott M. The athletic hernia: a systematic review. Clin Orthop Relat Res. 2007;455:78–87.

Ultrasound of hips and hernias by Marnix Van Holsbeeck. http://www.cme.umn.edu/prod/groups/med/@pub/@med/@cme/documents/content/med_content_256288.pdf.

Erik Adams

## Introduction

The use of ultrasound for injection guidance offers significant advantages over unguided injections and even over fluoroscopic guidance. Regarding the latter, ultrasound delivers no ionizing radiation, can be easily used in any clinical setting, and allows visualization of neurovascular structures, which could be harmed with a needle. Compared to unguided injections, ultrasound-guided injections are more accurate, and the clinician can undertake a wider variety of injections, which would otherwise be unsafe or simply impossible without guidance. However, ultrasound guidance has a steep learning curve, and for this reason, safety is not automatically guaranteed by the use of ultrasound guidance.

A crucial element of learning ultrasound guidance is the development of and adherence to proper procedures. Maintaining visualization of the needle is often difficult at first, and one may be tempted to fall back on techniques used for unguided injections, advancing the needle until it hits the target, all the while waiting for the needle to appear on the ultrasound screen. Combining this tendency with an appetite for trying new injections, one can see how safety may be compromised when injecting near lung, bowel, or larger arteries. For this reason, it is best to start with injections that are generally considered safe when unguided, such as the knee or the subacromial–subdeltoid (SASD) bursa of the shoulder, and develop competence with needle guidance before venturing into new territory. It is also recommended that injections be attempted on cadavers, with experienced instruction, before proceeding to inject the living.

E. Adams, MD, PhD (✉)
Midwest Sports Medicine Institute,
2521 Allen Boulevard, Middleton, WI 53562, USA
e-mail: erikadams@pol.net

## Accuracy of Ultrasound-Guided vs. Palpation-Guided Injections

A number of studies have investigated whether ultrasound guidance confers an improvement in the accuracy of injections into joints, bursae, and tendon sheaths. As shown in Table 15.1, ultrasound guidance typically results in a 100 % accuracy rate for most targets, whereas the accuracy of palpation-guided injections appears to be quite variable. Those studies that obtain a high degree of accuracy for unguided injections not surprisingly state that unguided is the method of choice, notwithstanding that not all studies have achieved similar results. The most obvious variable distinguishing each of these studies from each other, however, is the identity of the person performing the unguided injection. It is conceivable that the technique or experience of the individual performing an unguided injection is the greatest determinant of accuracy. Some physicians appear to be able to achieve 100 % accuracy with unguided injections in the SASD bursa or wrist, for example, but results such as these should not be construed to imply that everyone can do the same. A study [1] comparing injection accuracy when a rheumatology fellow was using ultrasound guidance and a rheumatology faculty member was using palpation guidance produced superior results, in fact, for the fellow.

Some targets appear to present a greater challenge to accuracy for unguided injections than others. The pes anserinus bursa showed a 92 % accuracy rate for ultrasound-guided injection of latex into cadaver specimens, compared to a 17 % rate for unguided [2]. What is remarkable about this study, however, is that in the control group, ultrasound guidance was used to identify landmarks and mark the skin. These were used to guide the injection [3]. One might expect an even worse result using blind technique with palpation only. Tendon sheaths appear to be similarly difficult, with inadvertent injection into the tendon a common occurrence for unguided injections. Unguided injections in cadaveric

J.M. Daniels and W.W. Dexter (eds.), *Basics of Musculoskeletal Ultrasound*,
DOI 10.1007/978-1-4614-3215-9_15, © Springer Science+Business Media New York 2013

**Table 15.1** Summary of studies on the accuracy of guided vs. unguided injections

| Reference | Target, patient type | Method of confirmation | Other | US-guided accuracy | Unguided accuracy |
|---|---|---|---|---|---|
| Muir et al. [10] | Peroneal tendon sheath, cadaver | Latex injection, dissection | | 100 % (20 of 20) | 60 % (12 of 20), four intra-tendinous |
| Rutten et al. [11] | SASD bursa, live patients | Gadolinium injection, MRI | | 100 % (10 of 10) | 100 % (10 of 10) |
| Hashiuchi et al. [12] | Long-head biceps tendon sheath, live patients | Contrast injection, CT | | 87 % (13 of 15) | 27 % (4 of 15) |
| Cunnington et al. [1] | Multiple large- to medium-sized joints, live patients | Contrast injection, X-ray | US-guided injections performed by fellow, unguided by faculty | 83 % (76 of 92) | 66 % (61 of 92) |
| Luz et al. [13] | Wrist, live patients | Contrast | "Wrist joint"—not further specified | 27 of 30 | 27 of 30 |
| Curtiss et al. [4] | Knee, cadaver | Latex injection, dissection | Comparison of more- vs. less-experienced injector | 100 % for both more and less experienced (20 injections each) | 100 % (20 of 20) more experienced / 55 % (11 of 20) less experienced |
| Khosla et al. [6] | Foot TMT joints, cadaver | Methylene blue injection, dissection | Fluoroscopic accuracy 89 % combined TMT joints 1 and 2 | 64 % combined TMT joints 1 and 2 (18 of 28) | 25 % combined TMT joints 1 and 2 (7 of 28)[a] |
| Sabeti-Aschraf et al. [14] | Acromioclavicular joint, cadaver | Ultrasound exam | Large volume injected, to aid detection | 95 % (54 of 57) | 72 % (31 of 43) |
| Finoff et al. [2] | Pes anserinus bursa, cadaver | Latex injection, dissection | Unguided injection used ultrasound to mark location | 92 % (11 of 12) | 17 % (2 of 12)—partially ultrasound-guided |
| Wisniewski et al. [8] | Ankle anterior joint line, cadaver | Latex injection, dissection | Long-axis approach | 100 % (20 of 20) | 85 % (17 of 20) |
| Wisniewski et al. [8] | Ankle sinus tarsi, cadaver | Latex injection, dissection | Short-axis approach | 90 % (18 of 20) | 35 % (7 of 20) |
| Reach et al. [15] | Ankle and foot structures, cadaver | Methylene blue, dissection | | 100 % (10 of 10) for first and second MTPJ, tibiotalar joint, FHL and tibia is posterior tendon sheaths. 90 % (9 of 10) for subtalar joint | Unguided injections not performed |
| Peck et al. [16] | Acromioclavicular joint, cadaver | Latex injection, dissection | | 100 % (10 of 10) | 40 % (4 of 10) |

[a]Ultrasound guidance technique unclear in this study

**Fig. 15.1** Arthroscopic photographs after unguided corticosteroid injections in the knee. (**a** and **b**) Lateral femoral condyle cratering with corticosteroid deposition in articular cartilage. (**c**) Needle skive mark (at 4 o'clock) and chondrolysis. (**d**) Inadvertent injection into ACL (photographs courtesy of Arthur Wardell, MD)

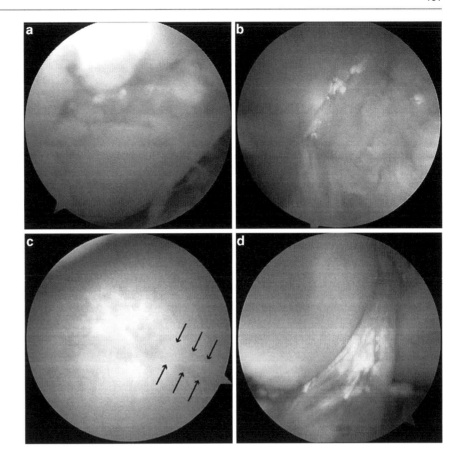

knees show a variable success rate, depending on experience, with a physician having almost 4 years of experience at unguided knee injections showing less success than a staff physician with 13 years' experience [4].

Injection accuracy with ultrasound guidance is, in most studies, superior to that with palpation guidance, but variable results are still observed with ultrasound guidance. This may be related to the experience of the physician. In the study cited above [1], the rheumatology fellow obtained a success rate of 83 % in ultrasound-guided injections, after 10 months' experience performing ultrasound-guided injections. A study of accuracy in ultrasound-guided sacroiliac joint injections showed an accuracy of 60 % for the first 30 injections performed by the investigator, then 94 % for the next 30 injections [5], again suggesting a learning curve.

Technique may play a substantial role in the accuracy of ultrasound-guided injections. In a study of injections into the foot's first and second tarsometatarsal joints [6], the combined accuracy for both joints was only 68 % using ultrasound guidance. This is substantially lower than other studies. A possible explanation may be that the author attempted to align the needle with the sagittal plane, rather than the coronal plane, the approach favored for this type of injection.

The issue of injection safety remains unaddressed in most of the studies regarding injection accuracy. A substantial concern is the potential for iatrogenic injury to articular cartilage, which likely would be irreversible. Figure 15.1 demonstrates intraoperative arthroscopic photographs of knee medial femoral condyle articular cartilage after recent blind corticosteroid injections. Full-thickness articular cartilage cratering (see Fig. 15.1a, b—In all pictures in this chapter, for the individual depicted as performing the procedures, the gloves are omitted for the sake of photographic clarity) has occurred, with corticosteroid embedded within the lesion. Linear needle skive marks found on articular cartilage (see Fig. 15.1c) result from sliding a needle between contacting articular surfaces. This concern for cartilage injury is applicable to any joint but is of particular significance to the knee, since the most reliable unguided injection portal is considered to be lateral mid-patellar (93 % accuracy [7]), which necessitates sliding the needle between the articular surfaces of the lateral patellar facet and lateral trochlear groove. Finally, the inadvertent injection of corticosteroid into the anterior cruciate ligament (ACL) (see Fig. 15.1d) should cast doubt on the advisability of injection into the notch of the knee, via the anterolateral portal.

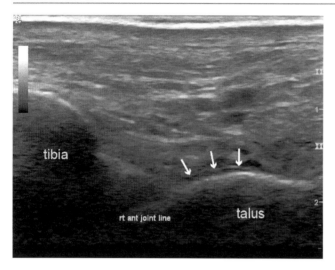

**Fig. 15.2** Talar dome articular cartilage is depicted by *arrows* and is vulnerable to needle trauma

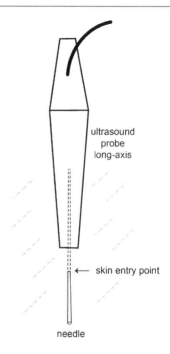

**Fig. 15.3** Depiction of needle placed long axis (also known as "in plane") under ultrasound probe

The articular surfaces of all diarthrodial joints should be considered to be vulnerable to injury during injection, so the ability to successfully enter the joint via unguided techniques should not be the only criterion for determining whether the use of ultrasound guidance is advisable. During ultrasound-guided injection of the talocrural joint of the ankle, for example, it is clear that the articular surface of the talar dome can be easily injured with the needle (Fig. 15.2). So while palpation-guided injection of this joint may be up to 100 % accurate [8], avoidance of potential articular cartilage injury by the use of ultrasound guidance should be a further consideration.

## Ultrasound Guidance: General Principles

Ultrasound-guided injections are more difficult than unguided injections, as the physician must add the additional tasks of maintaining an ideal sonographic image of the injection target, keeping the needle in view at all times, and steering the needle. Beginners should select injections that are typically easier. Ultrasound guidance also opens up a wide variety of deeper and more difficult injections that one would not attempt unguided, but many of these carry substantial risk for iatrogenic injury, such as perforation of large arteries, nerve trauma, and entry into the peritoneum or pleura.

It should be stressed that an injection is only directly ultrasound-guided if both the needle tip and the intended target are simultaneously in view. It is therefore possible to be using ultrasound during an injection but without true direct ultrasound guidance. Examples of this would include losing sight of the needle tip, having a poor or nonexistent image of the intended target, seeing the needle shaft but not the tip, or, when doing a short-axis injection, letting the needle tip proceed past the plane of the ultrasound beam.

When planning an ultrasound-guided injection, the intended needle tract should be examined with Doppler ultrasound for the presence of arteries, and consideration should also be given to the presence of nerves. Most injection targets can be approached by more than one route. Planning the injection should constitute a substantial portion of the time spent on the procedure. It is helpful to mark the planned needle trajectory on the skin and then sonographically examine this route, prior to putting a needle through it. If the needle tract passes close to an artery, the Doppler function should be used during needle advancement, until the needle tip passes the artery. It is also desirable to utilize a bony barrier to prevent needle penetration into underlying structures. For example, when injecting the psoas bursa, injecting at a point over the hip joint capsule carries a risk of entering the hip joint, and injecting too proximally carries the risk of entering the peritoneum. These concerns are addressed by injecting directly over the superior pubic ramus. Similarly, when injecting a costotransverse joint or the dorsal scapular nerve, staying over a rib prevents inadvertent needle entry into lung.

Once the needle approach to the target is chosen, then an optimized image of the intended target is obtained and maintained. The probe is then used as a guide for placement of the needle. Figure 15.3 illustrates this concept. When injecting long axis, the centerline of the probe defines a plane that extends down into the patient, and the needle is placed precisely along this plane. For this reason, one avoids looking at the ultrasound screen at first; the focus should be on the probe position, the plane of the ultrasound beam, and

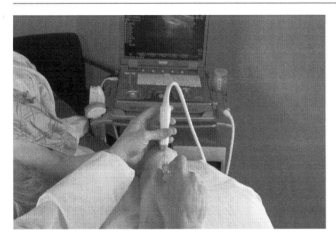

**Fig. 15.4** Alignment of needle probe, injection target, and ultrasound image

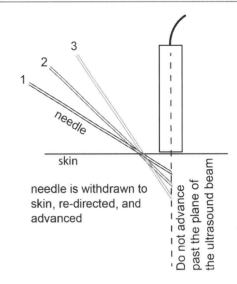

**Fig. 15.5** Short-axis (also known as "out of plane") injection technique depicting walking the needle tip deeper

angle needed to achieve the intended depth. Figure 15.4 demonstrates the proper arrangement of the physician, needle, probe, and screen. Note that they are colinear, which aids in placing the needle directly under the probe and only requires minimal movement of the eyes to look from the injection area to the screen.

Accurately placing a needle with a short-axis technique carries a different set of challenges. Once the optimized ultrasound image of the target is obtained and the probe is anchored to maintain that image, one has to construct a spatial correlation between the image on the screen and the position of the target under the probe. Many probes are marked at their center point, so it is best to center the intended target on the ultrasound screen, then use this center-point mark as a guide for needle placement. One should plan to intercept the plane of the ultrasound beam directly superficial to the intended target, then "walk" the needle down to the target. This is accomplished by withdrawing the needle and redirecting it at a steeper angle (Fig. 15.5). It is tempting to drive the needle deeper by pushing its tip past the plane of the ultrasound beam, but the needle tip is then entering unvisualized tissue, so the injection has become unguided at this point. When the needle tip reaches the plane of the ultrasound beam, it appears as a dot on the image, and it should not be advanced any further, unless, of course, one moves the probe farther from the needle entry point (Fig. 15.6).

Finally, one can use an oblique approach, which is sometimes helpful for avoiding arteries and nerves, and this is performed much as one does a short-axis technique. Whichever technique is chosen, the needle is initially inserted bevel up, which aids visualization of the needle tip with the ultrasound.

Typically, one advances the needle while injecting lidocaine, and then once in place, the syringe is changed and the desired therapeutic agent is injected. It is important not to move the needle while changing syringes. If a sterile ultra-

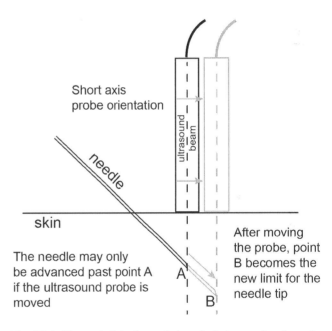

**Fig. 15.6** Short-axis injection technique depicting moving the probe so that needle can be safely advanced

sound probe cover is being used, the probe is laid onto the sterile field during this maneuver. If the probe is not sterile, it can be held by its cord by an assistant.

## Needle-Steering Techniques

The orientation of the needle bevel can be used to direct the needle. During advancement of the needle, the bevel acts as an inclined plane (Fig. 15.7). Additionally, the skin can be used as a fulcrum to steer the needle. Usually, both techniques are used simultaneously. If it is desired that the needle tip be brought more superficially, the bevel is placed down, and the needle is pressed into the skin to create an arc shape, which forces the needle tip more superficially. The opposite technique is used to deepen the needle tract (Fig. 15.8). This technique is useful for small adjustments in depth. When large adjustments are needed, it is best to withdraw the needle tip to the subcutaneous tissue and change the angle of entry.

## Sterile Technique

All injections should be done with aseptic technique, utilizing skin preparation with an antibacterial solution. If the probe is going to be close to the needle entry site, a sterile probe cover should be used for deeper injections, and for more superficial injections, the probe may also be sterilized with an antibacterial solution. Sterile ultrasound gel should also be used when the probe is close to the needle entry site. If a sterile probe cover is not used, the hand holding the probe is no longer sterile, which must be kept in mind. Breaches of sterile technique are common when learning ultrasound guidance.

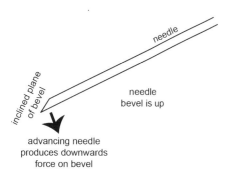

**Fig. 15.7** Effect of needle bevel on needle steering

## Patient Positioning

Minute changes in the position of the needle tip can make the difference between a successful and an unsuccessful ultrasound-guided injection. For this reason, the patient needs to be well stabilized. A seated position, for example, is only used if one is injecting the elbow, wrist, or hand, and the extremity is supported on a surface. It does not work well for a shoulder SASD bursa injection, as any swaying of the patient, however minimal, may move the needle out of the bursa.

## Platelet-Rich Plasma

Platelet-rich plasma (PRP) is often used for a variety of disorders of dense fibrous connective tissue, such as partial tendon tears, tendinosis, and partial ligament tears. Platelets contain a variety of growth factors, which makes them enticing for the treatment of chronic conditions, in which the healing process has halted. When treating tendinosis, the question arises as to how extensively the PRP should be distributed throughout the tendinopathic lesion. The issue is whether platelets freely diffuse within ground substance (the chief component within a tendinosis lesion) or among collagen fibers within a tendon.

This was investigated by the injection of PRP infiltrated with blue water-soluble dye into five cadaver Achilles tendons, either as a single aliquot or three aliquots; the tendon was then dissected, and the dye was found to have diffused over a median distance of 100 mm [9]. This was interpreted to mean that the platelets themselves diffused, supposedly justifying the use of this injection technique, as opposed to distributing the PRP evenly throughout a tendinosis lesion during the injection. However, this study did not actually demonstrate the diffusion of platelets but rather the diffusion of the blue dye, as detection of diffusion was performed by

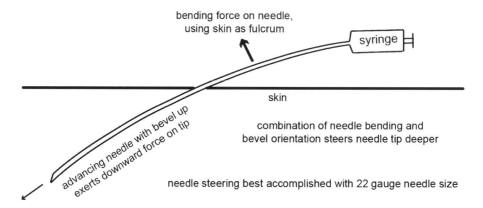

**Fig. 15.8** Needle-steering technique

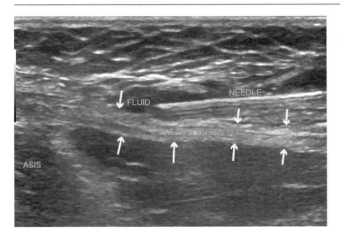

**Fig. 15.9** Hydrodissection of lateral femoral cutaneous nerve, depicted by *arrows*

visual inspection for the presence of blue color. Platelets are known to agglutinate immediately upon exposure to tissue, so their migration within a tendon is unlikely. Until there is definitive proof that platelets diffuse within tissue after being injected, the physician is encouraged to spend the extra effort to spread the PRP evenly throughout a tendinosis lesion.

## Hydrodissection

Fluid injection can be used to separate tissue planes or to create a space for injection of a therapeutic agent. For example, if two tissues pathologically adhere to each other, such as the median nerve and the flexor retinaculum at the wrist in carpal tunnel syndrome or a tendon and its sheath in teno-synovitis, the tissues are separated by hydrodissection, and then a corticosteroid can be injected between the two structures. Upon reaching the space to be hydrodissected, the needle bevel is turned down, and volume is injected as the needle is advanced (Fig. 15.9).

Nerve hydrodissection offers the opportunity to relieve peripheral nerve entrapment percutaneously. The technique involves injection of saline under the nerve sheath, briefly expanding the tissue circumferentially around the nerve. For very small nerves, such as the deep branch of the radial nerve within the arcade of Frohse, one cannot inject under the nerve sheath, so an attempt is made to hydrodissect the fibrous tissue in which the nerve resides. Since most nerves are accompanied by arteries, there is a potential not only for iatrogenic nerve injury, but also for arterial injury. At the very least, arterial injury will result in bleeding, which produces inflammation and fibrosis, perhaps resulting in re-entrapment of the nerve. At the very most, such as with nerves in the abdominal wall, arterial injury may not respond to the application of pressure. The approach to the nerve is always distal to the site of entrapment, and the probe should

image the nerve both longitudinally and transversely during needle advancement. When viewed short axis, the ideal position for the needle would be at the 12 o'clock position on the nerve. The bevel is turned down, and while injecting saline, the needle is advanced into the nerve sheath, then advanced along the sheath as it expands with saline. Typically, about 20 cm$^3$ are needed. Local anesthetic may be included if a diagnostic block is also desired. A successful nerve hydrodissection will show fluid surrounding the nerve circumferentially at the previous site of compression.

## Anesthesia

Injection of local anesthesia along the needle tract can be aided by ultrasound guidance, as sensitive tissues, such as fascia and synovium, can be visualized and injected prior to piercing them with the needle. However, it is also beneficial to learn a number of peripheral nerve blocks, especially when multiple needle approaches are planned, or extensive work is to be performed with the needle, such as when fenestrating a plantar aponeurosis origin. The use of a nerve block is also helpful when using PRP, as local anesthetic at the intended injection target may dilute the PRP more than is desirable. Nerve blocks can be performed by any physician that has developed skills at nerve hydrodissection, as the two techniques are similar.

## Injections by Joint

The tables included in this section illustrate the appropriate probe position, needle entry point, as well as the ultrasound image one should expect to obtain. Illustration of proper sterile technique (e.g., gloves, sterile prep, probe cover) has been omitted for the sake of clarity.

### Shoulder (Table 15.2)

#### Subacromial–Subdeltoid Bursa

Successfully completed, this injection will result in the symmetric expansion of the SASD bursa, which extends from the subacromial space to the deltoid insertion within the coronal plane and from the infraspinatus to the rotator interval in the sagittal plane. The expansion of the bursa, therefore, has a distinct appearance, which serves as confirmation of correct placement.

The patient is placed in the lateral decubitus position; a pillow is placed under the arm to relax the bursa. The probe is placed longitudinally along the supraspinatus, keeping the lateral acromion in view. The ultrasound screen is placed near the head of the bed. The needle approach is long axis.

**Table 15.2** Ultrasound-guided shoulder injections

| Target | Patient position | Ultrasound image | Pearls/pitfalls |
|---|---|---|---|
| SASD bursa | 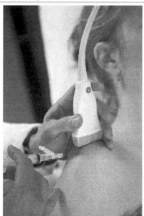Lateral decubitus | 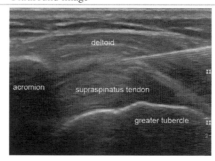 | Needle bevel down entering the bursa<br><br>Observe expansion of bursa in both the sagittal and coronal planes |
| AC joint | 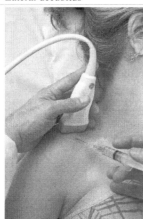Supine | 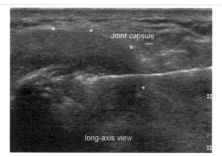 | Avoid hitting articular cartilage with needle<br><br>Use both long-axis and short-axis views<br><br>Joint capsule marked with asterisks in image at left |
| GH joint | 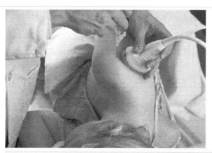Lateral decubitus | 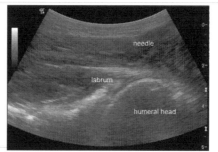 | Patient at edge of table, facing physician<br><br>Steep needle angle, tangential to humeral head<br><br>Bevel towards humeral head, slide under labrum |
| SC joint | 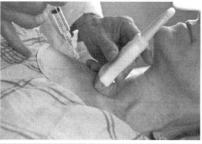Supine | 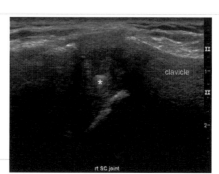 | For advanced practitioners only<br><br>Close proximity of blood vessels behind joint<br><br>Asterisk = needle short axis |

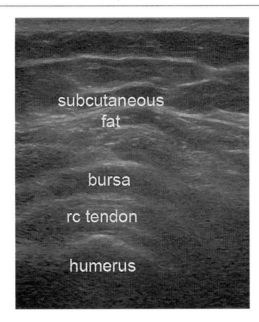

**Fig. 15.10** Short-axis view (probe in the sagittal oblique plane) of subacromial–subdeltoid bursa expansion with injection

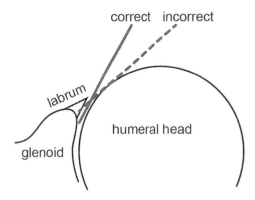

**Fig. 15.11** Tangential approach to the posterior glenohumeral joint

Upon reaching the bursa, the bevel is turned downwards, to avoid penetrating the paratenon with the needle tip. For difficult cases, such as an obese patient or a thickened peribursal fat layer, making the needle less visible, it may be helpful to turn the probe into the sagittal plane, once the needle is in place. The expansion of the bursa can be better appreciated sometimes with this view (Fig. 15.10). Keep in mind that in doing so, one needs to place the probe so that the plane of the ultrasound beam is at the tip of the needle. Slightly wiggling the needle can help with visualization. A test injection of lidocaine will confirm placement before injecting the desired therapeutic agent.

### Acromioclavicular Joint

The patient is supine, and the probe is turned into the patient's coronal plane, with the acromioclavicular (AC) joint centered. Note is made of the depth of the joint beneath the skin. Approach is from the anterior aspect, short axis to the probe, starting at a point on the skin that will result in the correct needle depth, when the needle is kept nearly parallel to the probe. While advancing the needle, it is helpful to turn the probe into the sagittal plane (long axis to the needle), to discern both the trajectory of the needle and its distance from the joint. As the needle penetrates the joint capsule, the probe is turned short axis, and the needle position can be adjusted to allow its placement within the "V" of the joint space. This avoids needle contact with articular cartilage.

### Glenohumeral Joint

This is the most difficult of the shoulder injections, as the needle trajectory is steep, the target is deep, and one must avoid penetrating the glenoid labrum. When this injection is performed with fluoroscopic guidance, it is more difficult to avoid the labrum. The patient is placed in the lateral decubitus position, rolled with the top shoulder, the side being injected, slightly towards the person performing the injection. This gives access to the posterior aspect of the shoulder. A curved low-frequency probe is preferred. The probe is placed into the axial plane, demonstrating the posterior humeral head and posterior labrum. The needle is inserted long axis, at an angle that is tangential to the humeral head, at the location of the labrum (Fig. 15.11). Upon reaching the space between the humeral head and labrum, the bevel is turned towards the humeral head, and while injecting lidocaine or saline, it is slid into the joint space. Injecting fluid during needle advancement will "float" the labrum slightly, lifting it out of the way.

When injecting an end-stage arthritic glenohumeral (GH) joint or frozen shoulder, it may be helpful to utilize the same needle entry point to block the suprascapular nerve (SSN) in the posterior glenoid fossa (see below).

### Sternoclavicular Joint

The sternoclavicular (SC) joint should only be injected with imaging guidance, never without, because of the presence of the carotid artery, deep to the joint. This is an advanced injection and should not be approached casually. The probe is first turned transversely across the joint, then turned 90°, placing the plane of the ultrasound beam directly in the center of the joint. This allows more careful monitoring of needle depth. Approach is from a point caudad to the probe, long axis. Once the joint is reached, the probe is turned short axis, to ensure that the needle tip is placed at the midpoint of the joint and is not touching articular cartilage. During the syringe change, care is taken to not advance the needle any deeper.

### Suprascapular Nerve Block (Not Shown in Table)

This injection may be useful for adhesive capsulitis of the shoulder, or as a diagnostic maneuver for suspected SSN entrapment. The SSN lies in the glenoid fossa at the posterior aspect of the shoulder. This location is visualized by first placing the probe transversely across the posterior joint line of the GH joint, then sliding it medially while turning the probe about 10–15° oblique, with the medial side of the probe more cephalad. The suprascapular artery can be identified with Doppler imaging, and the nerve is adjacent to this artery, against the cortex of the neck of the glenoid process. The patient's shoulder should be kept in internal rotation (hand on abdomen) to avoid filling the venous network alongside the suprascapular artery and nerve. Hydrodissecting the nerve away from the bone will lift the entire neurovascular bundle away from the needle tip, decreasing the likelihood of an arterial or venous puncture. Typically, a long-acting local anesthetic is used for the block, unless a brief duration block is desired for diagnostic purposes (suspected SSN entrapment).

## Elbow (Table 15.3)

### Medial or Lateral Epicondyle

With the use of ultrasound, it becomes apparent that many patients formerly diagnosed with epicondylitis have partial tears of the common flexor or extensor tendons at the medial or lateral epicondyles, respectively. When such tears are diagnosed, the use of corticosteroid becomes questionable, and one may want to resort to PRP or whole blood. The probe is laid longitudinally along the tendon, and the approach is from the distal aspect, long axis. The interior surface of the tear is repeatedly fenestrated, as is the denuded bone at the site of the tear, injecting during the fenestration.

### Cubital Tunnel

Entrapment of the ulnar nerve can occur within the cubital tunnel or more distally between the two heads of the flexor carpi ulnaris (FCU). A longitudinal sonographic view of the nerve may show an hourglass configuration to the nerve, at the site of the entrapment, and proximal to the entrapment, the cross-sectional area of the nerve will be increased. Hydrodissecting the nerve with saline may release it from its entrapment. The procedure outlined at the beginning of this section is applicable here.

## Wrist (See Table 15.3)

### Carpal Tunnel

Ultrasound guidance in carpal tunnel injections offers a multitude of benefits, including avoidance of inadvertent intra-tendinous or intraneural injection, assurance that the injection is actually deep to the flexor retinaculum of the wrist, as well as hydrodissecting the nerve away from the underside of the flexor retinaculum, if desired. The carpal tunnel is best approached distally but can also be approached from the ulnar side of the volar wrist. Whichever the approach, this should be considered an advanced injection.

The distal approach utilizes a short-axis orientation. The probe is placed transversely over the median nerve and the flexor retinaculum, keeping in mind that an injection proximal to the flexor retinaculum is not actually a carpal tunnel injection. Power Doppler is used to detect the presence of the uncommon median artery, as well as to detect any arteries along the intended needle tract. The probe is then centered at the ulnar edge of the median nerve. As with all short-axis injections, the initial placement of the needle should be superficial to its desired, final depth, and then withdrawn slightly and redirected deeper. As the needle passes through the flexor retinaculum, its bevel is turned downwards, and lidocaine is injected, so that any structures along the deep surface of the flexor retinaculum are pushed aside by the lidocaine. If the needle is at the ulnar edge of the nerve, this will hydrodissect the nerve away from the flexor retinaculum. The needle can be redirected towards the radial side of this new fluid space, and the hydrodissection can be carried across the full width of the needle. It is helpful to also visualize the distal aspect of the carpal tunnel, to ensure that the hydrodissection also extends distally. If not, and if it was apparent during initial hydrodissection that the nerve was adherent to the flexor retinaculum, a steeper needle angle will be needed to address the distal aspect of the carpal tunnel. Once satisfactory hydrodissection is completed, the syringe is changed, and corticosteroid is injected. This technique allows placement of the corticosteroid both around the swollen nerve and the underside of the thickened flexor retinaculum.

When utilizing an approach from the ulnar side of the wrist, it is extremely easy to pierce the ulnar artery. If the patient lacks sufficient forearm supination, placing the patient in a supine position with the arm overhead, supported on pillows, may be preferable. The probe is laid transversely over the carpal tunnel, and the needle approach is long axis. The median nerve and flexor retinaculum should be clearly visible. The needle trajectory should place the needle tip at the ulnar edge of the contact point between the nerve and retinaculum. As the needle passes through the flexor retinaculum, its bevel is turned downwards, and lidocaine is injected upon passing through, so as to avoid puncturing the nerve.

### First Dorsal Compartment (de Quervain's)

The aim of this injection is to place corticosteroid between the tendon pair within the first dorsal compartment (adductor pollicis longus and abductor pollicis brevis) and their shared tendon sheath. An intra-tendinous injection should be avoided. The patient is seated, facing the examiner. The probe is placed transversely over the first dorsal compartment, and the division between the two tendons is identified, keeping in mind that in chronic cases of de Quervain's tenosynovitis, there

**Table 15.3**  Ultrasound-guided elbow and wrist injections

| Target | Patient position | Ultrasound image | Pearls/pitfalls |
|---|---|---|---|
| Elbow, lateral epicondyle | | | If using PRP or whole blood, fenestrate tendon and bone at site of tear |
| | Seated alongside table | | Use lidocaine or saline to identify longitudinal tears |
| Cubital tunnel | | | Hydrodissect ulnar nerve at FCU if signs of entrapment |
| | Supine, arm overhead | Asterisk—constricted portion of ulnar nerve; hydrodissection has already been performed distally | Needle bevel down |
| | | | Begin hydrodissection distal to site of entrapment |
| First dorsal compartment of wrist | | | Branch of radial artery lies along deep surface of tendon sheath |
| | Seated alongside table | Arrow—needle short axis | Place needle between the two tendons within sheath |
| Carpal tunnel | | | If ulnar approach, avoid ulnar artery |
| | Seated alongside table (distal approach shown) | Arrow—needle short axis | If distal approach, aim for ulnar edge of median nerve |
| | | Median nerve highlighted with oval | |
| | | Calipers showing thickness of flexor retinaculum (1.2 mm) | Bevel down upon passing through flexor retinaculum |

may be longitudinal tendon splitting, making this identification difficult. The tendons should also be followed distally, as they may separate into separate tendon "slips" or separate compartments, which may need to be individually injected. Doppler imaging is used to identify the small branch of the radial artery, which lies at the deep surface of the tendon sheath. The approach is distal, short axis. Upon penetrating the tendon sheath, the bevel is turned downwards, and while injecting lidocaine, the needle tip is advanced, hydrodissecting the sheath away from the tendon pair. The hydrodissection should be continued until an approximately 3-cm long fluid space is created within the tendon sheath, prior to injecting corticosteroid.

### Thumb Carpometacarpal Joint (Not Shown in Table)

The thumb carpometacarpal (CMC) joint is frequently arthritic, and good relief can be obtained with a corticosteroid injection. The injection should avoid traumatizing the first dorsal compartment of the wrist and the branch of the radial artery that passes under this compartment. The probe is laid longitudinally along the joint, and the needle approach is short axis, aiming for the V-shaped notch in the joint. This should give a similar appearance as is shown in a midtarsal joint injection in Table 15.7.

### Hand (Not Shown in Table)

### MCP and IP Joints

These injections are performed short axis, with the probe placed longitudinally along the dorsal aspect of the joint. The proper digital arteries surround the joint, and these should be well visualized with Doppler imaging and marked on the skin. Since these constitute an end-arterial supply to the fingers, they must not be damaged, as an ischemic finger could possibly result. Ultrasound guidance allows avoidance not only of these arteries but also the articular cartilage. Successful needle placement should place the needle tip at the midpoint of the "V" shape of the joint space, deep to the synovium. Upon injection in the joint space, the synovium and capsule will be seen to rise.

### Trigger Finger

The aim of this injection is to place corticosteroid between the thickened A1 pulley in the distal palm and the flexor digitorum superficialis and profundus tendons (or just the flexor pollicis longus tendon, in the case of trigger thumb). Viewed transversely, the A1 pulley is usually scarcely visible, but in trigger finger, it appears as a thickened, hypoechogenic arc over the tendon pair (Fig. 15.12). The probe is placed over the A1 pulley, and the approach is from the distal aspect. The needle advancement is monitored both short axis and long axis. The needle bevel should be turned down,

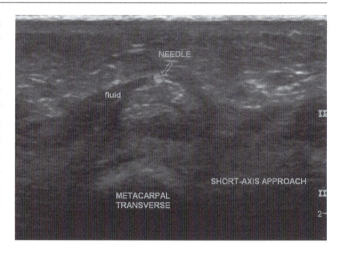

**Fig. 15.12** Trigger finger injection, short axis. Note the thickened A1 pulley

injecting lidocaine while advancing through the A1 pulley, in order to hydrodissect the pulley away from the tendon surface. This creates a space for the corticosteroid and ensures that the steroid is not being injected into either the tendon or A1 pulley. As tendon entrapment occurs at both the radial and ulnar aspects of the A1 pulley, the injection should be carried out at both sides of the tendon.

### Hip and Pelvis (Table 15.4)

### Hip Joint Capsule

Hip injections can be utilized diagnostically with local anesthetic, to distinguish between intra-articular and extra-articular pain generators and, therefore, pare down what is usually an extensive differential diagnosis, or therapeutically. Hip joint injections are actually intracapsular, as opposed to targeting the joint space itself. The hip capsule extends from the acetabulum, over the femoral head, and along the femoral neck, to a point just proximal to the intertrochanteric line, and then it reflects back on itself, to insert at a point approximately halfway down the femoral neck. For this reason, needle placement at the distal femoral neck has the potential to penetrate through both layers of the capsule at this location and, therefore, end up being extracapsular. The lateral femoral circumflex artery lies superficial to the femoral neck and should be identified by Doppler. The patient is placed supine, and the curved, low-frequency probe is placed along the axis of the femoral neck. After anesthetizing the skin, a long needle (typically 3.5 in.) is advanced long axis and guided around the lateral femoral circumflex artery, aiming for the junction between the femoral head and neck. Both the fascial plane containing the artery and the hip joint capsule are sensitive, so they should be well anesthetized before penetrating them with the needle tip. Once reaching the cortex

**Table 15.4**  Ultrasound-guided hip and pelvis injections

| Target | Patient position | Ultrasound image | Pearls/pitfalls |
|---|---|---|---|
| Hip capsule | Supine | Needle highlighted for clarity | Avoid lateral femoral circumflex artery<br><br>Contact point is junction of femoral head and neck |
| Sub-gluteus medius bursa | Lateral decubitus | | Posterior approach under tendon<br><br>Tendon should lift with injection<br><br>Bursa extends posteriorly |
| SI joint | Prone | Needle highlighted for clarity | Long-axis approach to superior SI joint<br><br>Note SI ligaments<br><br>Tilt probe to improve view of joint space |

of the femur, a test injection of 2 cm³ of sterile normal saline with 0.5 cm³ of air is helpful to confirm intracapsular placement; the bubble should pass over the anterior femoral head during the injection. Expansion of the joint capsule may also be seen, but keep in mind that with inadvertent placement of the needle tip deep to the reflected portion of the capsule (i.e., too distal), the capsule may appear to rise, but the injection is actually extracapsular. If possible, this injection may be performed on the X-ray table, and 1 cm³ of radiographic contrast material and a spot AP plain film can be used to confirm placement in difficult cases (Fig. 15.13).

## Sub-Gluteus Medius and Trochanteric Bursae

The sub-gluteus medius bursa, as its name implies, lies along the deep surface of the gluteus medius tendon, at the greater trochanter of the femur. The trochanteric bursa lies between the gluteus medius tendon and the iliotibial band, also over the greater trochanter. Both bursae can be injected from a posterior approach, long axis. The patient is in the lateral decubitus position, and the curved low-frequency probe is placed transversely across the greater trochanter, identifying the target structure. After anesthetizing skin, a long (typically 3.5 in.) needle is advanced into the bursa, anesthetizing the entire needle tract. A successful injection will see the overlying tendon lift.

## Psoas Bursa (Not Shown in Table)

The psoas bursa extends from anterior to the hip joint, where it communicates with that joint in approximately 30 % of cases, to the insertion of the iliopsoas tendon onto the lesser trochanter of the femur. As the iliopsoas curves over the anterior aspect of the hip joint, the bursa is under compression,

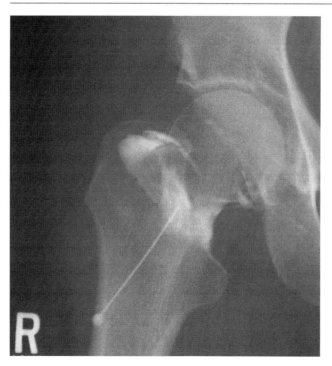

**Fig. 15.13** Plain-film hip arthrogram, showing needle in situ

approximately at the midline. One must keep in mind that the inclination of the sacrum requires that the probe be directed slightly caudad, if the ultrasound beam is to be in an orthogonal relationship to the bony cortex and thus produce a good image. This inclination of the probe makes it more difficult to place the needle within the middle of the ultrasound beam, so needle conspicuity is difficult for this injection. Because the PSIS overhangs the joint slightly, it is also difficult to see the inclination of the joint space and thus determine the appropriate inclination of the needle entry. In some patients, the joint space may be seen by heel-toeing the probe, directing it laterally, to shoot under the overhanging PSIS.

The longitudinal approach to the SI joint requires that the probe be centered in the joint longitudinally, and the needle is directed cephalad, long axis to the probe. The probe will be rotated about 10–15° with respect to the sagittal plane, to match the orientation of the SI joint. Whichever approach to the SI joint is used, transverse or longitudinal, once the needle is in the joint, one should be able to see the swirling of injectate within the joint with Doppler imaging, and this should be considered a normal part of the injection protocol.

so fluid collections are not typically seen at this location in cases of psoas bursitis, but rather more distally. However, the preferred injection location is over the superior pubic ramus, as the distal aspect of the bursa is much deeper and has overlying neurovascular structures. Injecting over the superior pubic ramus allows avoidance of the hip joint, hip labrum, and also peritoneum. However, the examiner must be capable of identifying and avoiding the structures of the inguinal canal, so this injection should only be attempted by experienced practitioners. The patient is placed supine, and the probe is oriented transversely over the superior pubic ramus, demonstrating the pectineus muscle medially, the iliopsoas over the lateral aspect of the bone, and the contents of the inguinal canal. The needle is advanced short axis down to the bone, then bevel turned down, and the injection should surround the tendon of the iliopsoas.

## Sacroiliac Joint

The sacroiliac joint (SI) may be approached transversely or longitudinally. Both are difficult and should be practiced repeatedly on a cadaver before attempting it on the living. For the transverse approach, the curved low-frequency ultrasound probe is placed transversely across the SI joint at the level of the posterior superior iliac spine (PSIS) and the S2 neural foramen, and the needle is long axis to the probe. The needle entry point will be medial to the probe position, moving farther to the contralateral side, the larger the patient. For a patient of normal body mass index, the needle will enter

## Knee (Table 15.5)

### Suprapatellar Recess

The suprapatellar recess route avoids any potential contact with articular cartilage or meniscus. When the patient has a small knee effusion, this injection is relatively easy, but when the knee is dry, it can be challenging. While visualizing the distal quadriceps femoris tendon longitudinally, the patient should be asked to perform an isometric quadriceps contraction, which will lift the tendon away from the suprapatellar recess and draw any joint fluid into the suprapatellar recess. Most patients have a small amount of intra-articular fluid, so some small area of fluid can usually be localized by this method. The patient is supine for the injection, knee either fully extended or flexed no more than about 15°. The probe is first placed longitudinally over the quadriceps tendon, to identify structures and any potential fluid space to target, then turned transversely. The approach is from the lateral side, long axis. When the knee is dry, the suprapatellar recess will need to be opened with lidocaine or saline, and it can be difficult to find the appropriate layer. A successful injection will demonstrate the suprapatellar recess opening symmetrically, usually demonstrating a bow-tie shape, along the deep surface of the quadriceps tendon. Care should be taken to not inject too distally, in the area of the suprapatellar fat pad, as the suprapatellar recess extends along the deep surface of this fat pad and is sometimes difficult to identify this far caudad.

**Table 15.5**  Ultrasound-guided knee injections

| Target | Patient position | Ultrasound image | Pearls/pitfalls |
|---|---|---|---|
| Knee joint (suprapatellar recess) | <br>Supine | | Injection in obese knee illustrated<br><br>Needle parallel to probe<br>Symmetric expansion of suprapatellar recess<br>Monitor injection in longitudinal axis also |
| Pes anserine bursa | <br>Supine, hip externally rotated | | Avoid branch of saphenous artery and vein, adjacent to bone<br><br>Consider saphenous nerve branch entrapment |

## Prepatellar Bursa (Not Shown in Table)

This relatively simple injection can be approached from any angle, long or short axis. In acute cases of prepatellar bursitis, identification of the bursa is straightforward, but in chronic cases, the bursa may contain hypertrophied synovium and little fluid. Doppler imaging may be utilized to distinguish synovitis from an effusion, as the former will show hyperemia. Test injections of lidocaine may be needed to confirm opening of the bursa, to ensure correct placement. Since the bursa is very superficial in patients of normal weight, care should be taken to not penetrate the ultrasound probe with the needle. It may be helpful to briefly lift the probe away from the skin during initial needle advancement, then place the probe back on the skin to access the needle trajectory.

## Pes Anserinus Bursa

The pes bursa lies between the pes anserinus tendon group and the medial cortex of the proximal tibia. One may approach this from the distal aspect, which requires traversing the tendons, or approaching anteriorly, sliding under the anterior margins of the tendon. The former approach is the easier of the two, but the latter approach avoids iatrogenic injury to tendon and is more comfortable. The saphenous artery and vein should be identified by Doppler, as they are adjacent to the bursa. The patient is placed supine, with the hip on the involved side externally rotated, to expose the anteromedial tibia. The probe is placed longitudinally along the distal pes tendons, and needle entry is distal to the probe, long axis. A successful injection should see expansion of the bursa and lifting of the tendons. The patient may not have pes anserine bursitis, if the exam fails to demonstrate fluid in the bursa. Branches of the saphenous nerve can become entrapped between the pes tendons or in the distal aspect of the medial collateral ligament.

## Ankle (Table 15.6)

## Talocrural Joint

Blind injections of the ankle talocrural joint risk iatrogenic injury to the talar dome articular cartilage, as does a poorly performed guided injection. The needle must be oriented tangential to that cartilage. The probe is placed longitudinally over the joint and the articular cartilage identified. Overlying tendons and the dorsalis pedis artery are also

**Table 15.6** Ultrasound-guided ankle injections

| Target | Patient position | Ultrasound image | Pearls/pitfalls |
|---|---|---|---|
| Ankle anterior joint line | 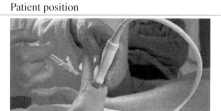<br>Semi-recumbent, hip and knee flexed | 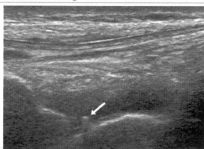 | Avoid articular cartilage of talus by directing slightly cephalad<br><br>Avoid overlying tendons and dorsalis pedis artery (see photo for mark on skin) |
| Ankle posterior joint line | 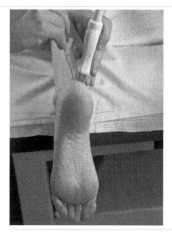<br>Prone, foot off table | 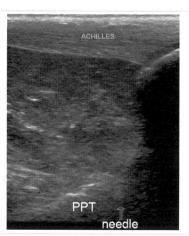<br>Short-axis approach | For posterior impingement<br><br>Probe longitudinal over Achilles<br>Needle approach is oblique to probe<br>Enter lateral to Achilles, steep angle<br>PPT = posterior process of talus |
| Ankle tendon sheath | 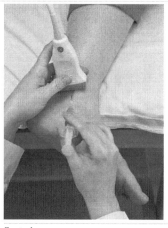<br>Seated | 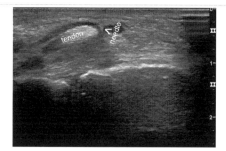<br>Tibialis posterior tendon distal to medial malleolus illustrated | Contact tendon bevel down<br><br>Injectate should surround tendon<br>Use adequate volume to expand sheath |

identified and can be marked on the skin with indelible ink. The probe is placed longitudinally over the joint line. A long-axis approach [8] from the distal aspect simplifies the task of avoiding overlying tendon and arterial structures, but not all patients are able to adequately plantar flex their ankle. In addition, the shallow needle angle that this approach affords may not allow the needle tip to be placed deep to the synovium. A short-axis approach is therefore preferred, but the needle needs to be directed at a slightly cephalad angle, to avoid pointing it at the articular cartilage of the talar dome. Also, the needle's path through overlying tissue must be observed at every tendon and artery, as it descends to the joint, to ensure that these are not being penetrated. Once the needle tip is deep to the synovium of the joint, injection should lift the synovium and joint capsule.

### Tendon Sheath Injection

Most of the tendons of the ankle joint are invested with tendon sheaths, as they follow a curved course. These tendon sheaths are susceptible to developing tenosynovitis. In acute cases, there will likely be fluid surrounding the tendon, making injection guidance much easier. In chronic cases, the tendon sheath will be thickened and possibly adherent to the tendon, so it must be hydrodissected free of the tendon before injection of corticosteroid. The approach is typically from the distal aspect of the tendon, and the probe is turned both short axis and long axis to monitor the needle position. The needle tip should never enter the tendon. If hydrodissecting the tendon sheath free of the tendon, the bevel is turned down, and volume is injected while passing through the sheath. Upon reaching the potential space between sheath and tendon, the space will expand, and the needle can be advanced into that fluid space, carrying the hydrodissection proximally. A successful injection will show fluid placed circumferentially around the tendon.

### Tarsal Tunnel (Not Shown in Table)

Tarsal tunnel syndrome results from compression of the tibial nerve in the tarsal tunnel. An ultrasound exam should discern the presence of masses within this space, such as a ganglion cyst, or swollen tendons. Injection can target such pathology; the injection can be placed freely within the tarsal tunnel. In this case, ultrasound guidance allows assurance that the injectate is placed deep to the flexor retinaculum and not within a tendon or the tibial nerve. The relevant structures are identified sonographically, with the probe placed transversely over the tarsal tunnel. The needle should enter between the flexor digitorum longus (FDL) tendon and the neurovascular bundle. Care should be taken to not inject too distally, as the tibial nerve bifurcates into the medial and lateral plantar nerves, which course anteriorly within the tarsal tunnel and may be contacted posterior to the FDL tendon.

## Foot (Table 15.7)

### Plantar Aponeurosis

Plantar fasciopathy typically appears sonographically as a thickened and hypoechogenic plantar aponeurosis at its origin. When corticosteroid is used, this injection is placed along the deep surface of the plantar aponeurosis, as close to the origin as possible. When properly placed, the injectate should lift the plantar aponeurosis away from the calcaneus. The patient is placed in a prone position, with feet just off the end of the exam table. The plantar aponeurosis is first imaged longitudinally, and the distal end of its origin is centered on the screen. The probe is then rotated transversely, and the needle approach is long axis from the lateral side of the foot. Some patients may exhibit substantial sensitivity at the lateral side of their foot, so even anesthetizing that area may be difficult for them; a distal sural nerve block may be helpful in such cases. Extravasation of corticosteroid into the plantar fat pad may cause fat pad atrophy and iatrogenic heel pain, so needle placement must be exact, and the injectate volume should not exceed approximately 1 mL.

When injecting PRP into the plantar aponeurosis, the approach is longitudinal to the aponeurosis, long axis to the probe, and a tibial nerve block is necessary. Without this block, the patient will not be able to tolerate the multiple needle passes that are necessary to spread the PRP throughout the hypoechogenic area of the aponeurosis. PRP may also be used for partial tears of the plantar aponeurosis, which typically occur about 2 cm distal to its origin on the calcaneus. The needle approach is also long axis, longitudinally along the aponeurosis.

### Midtarsal or MTP Joint

The dorsalis pedis artery should be located and marked on the skin with indelible ink for a midtarsal joint injection, and for an MTP joint injection, the digital arteries should be located and marked, especially since these are end-arterial supplies for the toes. That is, damage to these arteries can result in ischemia to a toe, so despite the apparent benign nature of this injection, it is not for beginners. For any mid-tarsal or MTP joint, the probe is laid longitudinally along the dorsal aspect of the joint, and the needle approach is short axis. Whether to approach from the medial or lateral side depends on the presence of vulnerable structures. As always, the needle tip should not contact articular cartilage, and it must be deep to the synovium to be considered intra-articular.

### Morton's Neuroma

Morton's neuroma can be seen extruding from between the plantar surfaces of the metatarsal (MT) heads upon squeezing the foot at the level of the MT heads (Gauthier's test). The approach is usually from the plantar and distal aspect of the foot, although some may be best approached from the

**Table 15.7** Ultrasound-guided foot injections

| Target | Patient position | Ultrasound image | Pearls/pitfalls |
|---|---|---|---|
| Plantar aponeurosis | Prone, foot off table | Needle viewed short axis | Short-axis approach illustrated |
| | | | Needle tip at inferior surface of aponeurosis, close to calcaneus |
| | | | Aponeurosis should lift with injection |
| Morton's neuroma | Supine | Short-axis approach | Plantar foot very sensitive; consider tibial nerve block |
| | | Labeled structures | Use dorsal approach if neuroma located more dorsally |
| | | Arrow—needle | |
| | | MT—metatarsal | |
| Midtarsal joint | Seated on table, hip and knee flexed | | Avoid dorsalis pedis artery |
| | | | Consider steeper approach for avoiding tendons |
| | | | Needle should be deep to synovium |

dorsal side. A combination of long-axis and short-axis views should be utilized, to place corticosteroid circumferentially around the neuroma. When the mass is seen to be compressible, however, this may represent a bursitis, and corticosteroid may be deposited directly within the bursa. Consideration should be given to a tibial nerve block if injecting from the plantar side, as the toe interspaces are extremely sensitive.

## Atypical Injections

Once good needle guidance skills and safety habits are learned, one may attempt injections that might be considered atypical, in that they do not constitute a standard approach to a joint, bursa, or tendon sheath. Examples might be an injection at a tendon origin or insertion, a nerve entrapment that has created a trigger point, or a tissue that has been aggravated by a degenerative osteophyte. In planning such an injection, a thorough understanding of the relevant anatomy is essential, as well as adequate visualization of nearby nerves and blood vessels. In these situations, one must be competent with long axis, short axis, and oblique approaches, so that all options can be entertained and the safest route chosen. Whenever injecting the shoulder or torso, one must remain cognizant of the potential for entering pleura or peritoneum. In many cases, it is possible to plan the injection so that a bony backdrop, such as rib, prevents the needle from entering vital structures, should it be advanced too far.

## Summary

Ultrasound needle guidance creates for the physician a higher degree of injection accuracy, potentially a greater degree of safety, and also the possibility of performing injections of targets that could not be reached unguided. Ultrasound guidance has its own skill set, which should not be overlooked by those eager to apply this technique. One is encouraged to learn in a programmed environment with injections on cadavers and to realize that guided injections are more difficult to perform than unguided injections. To be successful, it is required that a high-quality image of the injection target be maintained throughout the injection, while the needle tip is kept in view whenever it is being advanced. Good safety practices include the use of aseptic technique, scanning with power Doppler to detect arteries along the needle tract, sonographically identifying all structures near the needle, avoiding moving the needle during syringe change, and planning the injection to prevent inadvertent needle entry into vital structures. This last point bears emphasis, as many factors can compromise safety in this regard, including a nervous or immature patient who cannot hold still or an obese patient in whom it is difficult to see both the injection target and the needle. It must be realized that, since the use of ultrasound guidance opens up many new possibilities for novel types of injections, the excitement this generates may encourage us to attempt procedures in situations that are intrinsically unsafe. In short, just because we can perform a procedure does not mean that we should. First, do no harm.

## References

1. Cunnington J, Marshall N, Hide G, Bracewell C, Isaacs J, Platt P, et al. A randomized, double-blind, controlled study of ultrasound-guided corticosteroid injection into the joint of patients with inflammatory arthritis. Arthritis Rheum. 2010;62(7):1862–9.
2. Finnoff JT, Nutz DJ, Henning PT, Hollman JH, Smith J. Accuracy of ultrasound-guided versus unguided pes anserinus bursa injections. PM R. 2010;2(8):732–9.
3. Bianchi S, Zamorani MP. In: Bianchi S, Martinoli C, editors. Ultrasound-Guided Interventional Procedures. Berlin: Springer; 2007. p. 892.
4. Curtiss HM, Finnoff JT, Peck E, Hollman J, Muir J, Smith J. Accuracy of ultrasound-guided and palpation-guided knee injections by an experienced and less-experienced injector using a superolateral approach: a cadaveric study. PM R. 2011;3(6):507–15.
5. Pekkafahli MZ, Kiralp MZ, Basekim CC, Silit E, Mutlu H, Oztürk E, et al. Sacroiliac injections performed with sonographic guidance. J Ultrasound Med. 2003;22(6):553–9.
6. Khosla S, Thiele R, Baumhauer JF. Ultrasound guidance for intra-articular injections of the foot and ankle. Foot Ankle Int. 2009;30(9):886–90.
7. Jackson DW, Evans NA, Thomas BM. Accuracy of needle placement into the intra-articular space of the knee. J Bone Joint Surg Am. 2002;84-A(9):1522–7.
8. Wisniewski SJ, Smith J, Patterson DG, Carmichael SW, Pawlina W. Ultrasound-guided versus nonguided tibiotalar joint and sinus tarsi injections: a cadaveric study. PM R. 2010;2(4):277–81.
9. Wiegerinck JI, Reilingh ML, de Jonge MC, van Dijk CK, Kerkhoffs GM. Injection techniques of platelet-rich plasma into and around the Achilles tendon. Am J Sports Med. 2011;39(8):1681–6.
10. Muir JJ, Curtiss HM, Hollman J, Smith J, Finnoff JT. The accuracy of ultrasound-guided and palpation-guided peroneal tendon sheath injections. Am J Phys Med Rehabil. 2011;90(7):564–71.
11. Rutten MJ, Collins JM, Maresch BJ, Smeets JH, Janssen CM, Kiemeney LA, et al. Glenohumeral joint injection: a comparative study of ultrasound and fluoroscopically guided techniques before MR arthrography. Eur Radiol. 2009;19(3):722–30.
12. Hashiuchi T, Sakurai G, Morimoto M, Komei T, Takakura Y, Tanaka Y. Accuracy of the biceps tendon sheath injection: ultrasound-guided or unguided injection? A randomized controlled trial. J Shoulder Elbow Surg. 2011;20(7):1069–73.
13. Luz KR, Furtado RNV, Nunes ICCG, Rosenfeld A, Fernandes ARC, Natour J. Ultrasound-guided intra-articular injections in the wrist in patients with rheumatoid arthritis: a double-blind, randomised controlled study. Ann Rheum Dis. 2008;67(8):1198.
14. Sabeti-Aschraf M, Lemmerhofer B, Lang S, Schmidt M, Funovics PT, Ziai P, et al. Ultrasound guidance improves the accuracy of the acromioclavicular joint infiltration: a prospective randomized study. Knee Surg Sports Traumatol Arthrosc. 2011;19(2):292–5.
15. Reach JS, Easley ME, Chuckpaiwong B, Nunley II JA. Accuracy of ultrasound guided injections in the foot and ankle. Foot Ankle Int. 2009;30(3):239–42.
16. Peck E, Lai JK, Pawlina W, Smith J. Accuracy of ultrasound-guided versus palpation-guided acromioclavicular joint injections: a cadaveric study. PM R. 2010;2(9):817–21.

## Suggested Reading

Checa A, Chun W, Pappu R. Ultrasound-guided diagnostic and therapeutic approach to Retrocalcaneal Bursitis. J Rheumatol. 2011;38(2): 391–2.
Chen CP, Lew HL, Tsai WC, Hung YT, Hsu CC. Ultrasound-guided injection techniques for the low back and hip joint. Am J Phys Med Rehabil. 2011;90(10):860–7.
Choudur HN, Ellins ML. Ultrasound-guided gadolinium joint injections for magnetic resonance arthrography. J Clin Ultrasound. 2011;39(1):6–11.
Collins JM, Smithuis R, Rutten MJ. US-guided injection of the upper and lower extremity joints. Eur J Radiol. 2012;81(10):2759–70.
Elkousy H, Gartsman GM, Drake G, Sola W Jr, O'Connor D, Edwards TB. Retrospective comparison of freehand and ultrasound-guided shoulder steroid injections. Orthopedics. 2011;34(4):270.

Finnoff JT, Hurdle MF, Smith J. Accuracy of ultrasound-guided versus fluoroscopically guided contrast-controlled piriformis injections: a cadaveric study. J Ultrasound Med. 2008;27(8):1157–63.

Gilliland CA, Salazar LD, Borchers JR. Ultrasound versus anatomic guidance for intra-articular and periarticular injections: a systematic review. Phys Sportsmed. 2011;39(3):121–31.

Hashiuchi T, Sakurai G, Sakamoto Y, Takakura Y, Tanaka Y. Comparative survey of pain-alleviating effects between ultrasound-guided injection and blind injection of lidocaine alone in patients with painful shoulder. Arch Orthop Trauma Surg. 2010;130(7):847–52.

Hartung W, Ross CJ, Straub R, Feuerbach S, Schölmerich J, Fleck M, et al. Ultrasound-guided sacroiliac joint injection in patients with established sacroiliitis: precise IA injection verified by MRI scanning does not predict clinical outcome. Rheumatology (Oxford). 2010;49(8):1479–82.

Hurdle MF, Wisniewski SJ, Pingree MJ. Ultrasound-guided intra-articular knee injection in an obese patient. Am J Phys Med Rehabil. 2012;91(3):275–6.

Kayhan A, Gökay NS, Alpaslan R, Demirok M, Yılmaz , Gökçe A. Sonographically guided corticosteroid injection for treatment of plantar fasciosis. J Ultrasound Med. 2011;30(4):509–15.

Lee DH, Han SB, Park JW, Lee SH, Kim KW, Jeong WK. Sonographically guided tendon sheath injections are more accurate than blind injections: implications for trigger finger treatment. J Ultrasound Med. 2011;30(2):197–203.

Mandl P, Naredo E, Conaghan PG, D'Agostino MA, Wakefield RJ, Bachta A, et al. Practice of ultrasound-guided arthrocentesis and joint injection, including training and implementation, in Europe: results of a survey of experts and scientific societies. Rheumatology (Oxford). 2012;51(1):184–90.

Mulvaney SW. Ultrasound-guided percutaneous neuroplasty of the lateral femoral cutaneous nerve for the treatment of meralgia paresthetica: a case report and description of a new ultrasound-guided technique. Curr Sports Med Rep. 2011;10(2):99–104.

Peck E, Finnoff JT, Smith J, Curtiss H, Muir J, Hollman JH. Accuracy of palpation-guided and ultrasound-guided needle tip placement into the deep and superficial posterior leg compartments. Am J Sports Med. 2011;39(9):1968–74.

Sabeti-Aschraf M, Ochsner A, Schueller-Weidekamm C, Schmidt M, Funovics PT, V Skrbensky G, et al. The infiltration of the AC joint performed by one specialist: ultrasound versus palpation a prospective randomized pilot study. Eur J Radiol. 2010;75(1):e37–40.

Sibbitt Jr WL, Peisajovich A, Michael AA, Park KS, Sibbitt RR, Band PA, et al. Does sonographic needle guidance affect the clinical outcome of intraarticular injections? J Rheumatol. 2009;36(9):1892–902.

Smith J, Finnoff JT, Levy BA, Lai JK. Sonographically guided proximal tibiofibular joint injection: technique and accuracy. J Ultrasound Med. 2010;29(5):783–9.

Smith J, Hurdle MF, Weingarten TN. Accuracy of sonographically guided intra-articular injections in the native adult hip. J Ultrasound Med. 2009;28(3):329–35.

Smith J, Finnoff JT, Santaella-Sante B, Henning T, Levy BA, Lai JK. Sonographically guided popliteus tendon sheath injection: techniques and accuracy. J Ultrasound Med. 2010;29(5):775–82.

Smith J, Wisniewski SJ, Finnoff JT, Payne JM. Sonographically guided carpal tunnel injections: the ulnar approach. J Ultrasound Med. 2008;27(10):1485–90.

Soh E, Li W, Ong KO, Chen W, Bautista D. Image-guided versus blind corticosteroid injections in adults with shoulder pain: a systematic review. BMC Musculoskelet Disord. 2011;12:137.

Ucuncu F, Capkin E, Karkucak M, Ozden G, Cakirbay H, Tosun M, et al. A comparison of the effectiveness of landmark-guided injections and ultrasonography guided injections for shoulder pain. Clin J Pain. 2009;25(9):786–9.

Yoong P, Guirguis R, Darrah R, Wijeratna M, Porteous MJ. Evaluation of ultrasound-guided diagnostic local anaesthetic hip joint injection for osteoarthritis. Skeletal Radiol. 2012;41(8):981–5.

Zufferey P, Revaz S, Degailler X, Balague F, So A. A controlled trial of the benefits of ultrasound-guided steroid injection for shoulder pain. Joint Bone Spine. 2012;79(2):166–9.

# Rheumatologic Findings

Ralf G. Thiele

## Approach to the Joint

### Description

For the assessment of rheumatic problems that involve the hand, wrist, or elbow, the patient will typically sit on a regular chair, at an examination table or a desk, across from the examiner [2]. The upper extremity can be placed on a cushion. This provides patient comfort and allows the examiner to slightly manipulate or maneuver the examined joint. For the assessment of rheumatic shoulder conditions, both patient and examiner can sit on rotating stools with wheels. For the ultrasound assessment of the lower extremity, the patient is typically placed prone or supine on the exam table. An assistant can help if the leg needs to be held in a certain position for a prolonged period of time.

### Probe Selection

When assessing rheumatic problems, the highest-frequency linear probe available should be used. Typically, we use frequencies between 12 and 18 MHz. Small footprint probes, or "hockey stick" probes, are not a necessary requirement but can be used for the assessment of small finger joints or structures near the medial or lateral malleolus of the ankle. Curvilinear probes are occasionally used in rheumatology if deeper-seated structures or obese patients are scanned. This can be particularly helpful for assessment of hip effusions and hip injections.

Since rheumatic conditions often involve inflammation of tissues, a sensitive Doppler function is essential. Power Doppler assesses the strength, or power, of blood flow. Color

R.G. Thiele, M.D. (✉)
Division of Allergy/Immunology and Rheumatology,
Department of Medicine, University of Rochester,
601 Elmwood Avenue, Box 695, Rochester, NY 14642, USA
e-mail: Ralf_thiele@urmc.rochester.edu

Doppler ultrasound encodes the direction of flow with variable colors. In rheumatology, the presence or absence, as well as the strength, of blood flow in inflamed tissues is of interest—the direction generally plays no role. For this reason, power Doppler is often chosen. With newer machines, color Doppler can be just as sensitive for the detection of flow. The examiner should try both modalities and choose the more sensitive one.

### Specific Presets

If possible, the use of machine presets for each specific joint should be used. These technical presets typically include frequency, depth, and focal points. If presets are not available, select the highest frequency that the probe can deliver. Adjustments may need to be made for the deeper-seated elbow, shoulder, and hip joints in obese patients.

Assessment of inflamed tissues is of great interest in rheumatic diseases. Color and power Doppler ultrasound can help appreciate normal and abnormal blood flow. Knowledge of physiologic vascularity is important for the appreciation of hyperemia in inflammation. Doppler signals that indicate blood flow need to be reliably distinguished from artifacts. If a particular tissue or area is identified in gray-scale (normal settings) ultrasound first, this tissue can then be examined with Doppler ultrasound for the presence of increased blood flow. The area of Doppler flow can be "matched" with an area of gray-scale ultrasound abnormalities. If a Doppler signal is seen over an area that makes no anatomic sense (e.g., a Doppler signal deep to the bony cortex, where sound waves are not reaching), this signal should be ignored. A Doppler signal that is pulsating synchronous with the pulse, and that makes anatomic sense, is likely to be a real signal. Fleeting Doppler signals that appear at random places are likely artifacts and should also be ignored. Decreasing the Doppler gain until artifacts deep to the bony cortex disappear can help find the balance between sensitivity and specificity.

## Common Problems

Finding the etiology of joint swelling is a common problem in rheumatology. History and physical examination can be helpful, but may not always help distinguish involvement of subcutaneous tissue, tendons, ligaments, or joints [3]. A swollen extremity or joint may be due to subcutaneous edema, tenosynovitis, synovitis, or injury. Conventional radiography is often used, but cannot demonstrate soft-tissue changes well. Ultrasound can provide detailed information about proliferative synovial tissue and fluid collections in tendon sheaths and joints, synovial hyperemia, bony erosions, enthesitis, and crystal deposits in gout or chondrocalcinosis [1].

will not be successful. If synovial hyperemia is detected, treatment for inflammatory arthritis can be considered, or a referral planned.

In a healthy joint, synovial tissue is usually not seen sonographically, as the synovial lining is only 1–3 cell layers strong [4]. Proliferative synovial tissue, the hallmark of inflammatory arthritis, typically has a hypoechoic sonographic appearance. It is interposed between hyperechoic, fibrous joint capsule, anechoic hyaline cartilage, and hyperechoic bony contour. Synovial fluid often has an anechoic (or "black") appearance. Fluid is displaceable with transducer pressure, while synovial tissue is slightly compressible but not displaceable.

### Synovitis (Fig. 16.1a, b)

Distension of the joint capsule by proliferation of synovial tissue or increased secretion of synovial fluid is here called synovitis.

Without the availability of soft-tissue imaging, joint swelling by any cause is often called synovitis. High-frequency ultrasonography allows one to distinguish effusion, synovial proliferation, and synovial hyperemia. This distinction can be important for diagnostic or therapeutic purposes. If fluid is detected, it can be aspirated for diagnostic purposes. If only synovial tissue is detected, an aspiration

### Tenosynovitis (Fig. 16.2)

Tenosynovitis is identified by distension of the tendon sheath by fluid or synovial tissue. Tenosynovitis is particularly common in wrists and ankles, where tendons are subjected to increased mechanical stress between bones and retinacula. The fibrous tendon sheath is lined with a delicate layer of synovial tissue, and the tendon itself is covered with an additional layer of synovial tissue. These two synovial layers are connected by the mesotendineum. Blood supply to the tendon body itself also runs through this tissue connector. In inflammatory arthritis and tenosynovitis, this synovial tissue thickens and fills the space

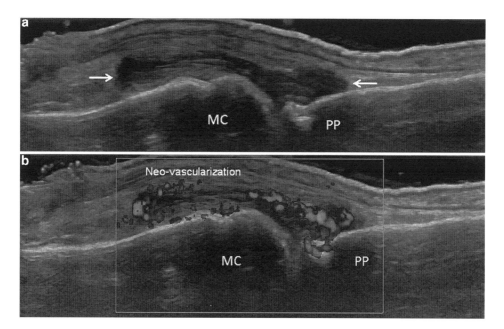

**Fig. 16.1** Metacarpophalangeal joint, dorsal long-axis view. Rheumatoid arthritis. Distension of the joint capsule by hypoechoic (*gray*) synovial tissue and anechoic (*black*) synovial fluid is seen between *arrows* ((**a**) *top*). Addition of power Doppler ((**b**) *bottom*) shows hyperemia of synovial tissue. Areas of neovascularization appear red orange under Doppler. *MC* metacarpal head; *PP* proximal phalanx

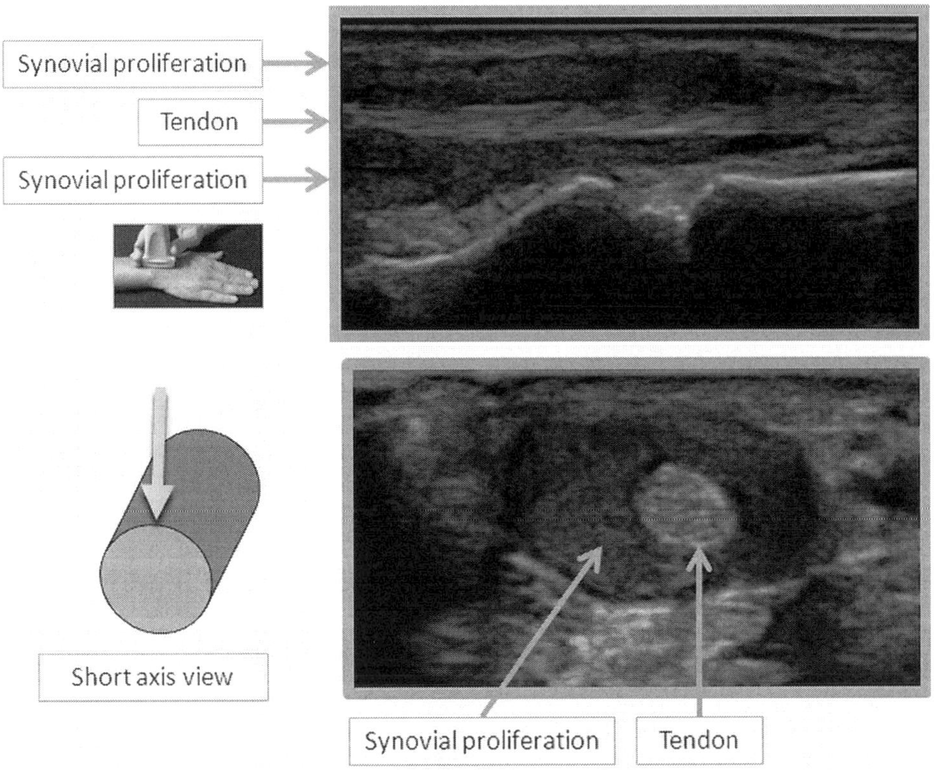

Synovial proliferation

Tendon

Synovial proliferation

Short axis view

Synovial proliferation     Tendon

**Fig. 16.2** Tenosynovitis. Chronic foreign-body reaction after wood splinter entered dorsal wrist. Long-axis view over dorsal wrist (*top*); short-axis view (*bottom*)

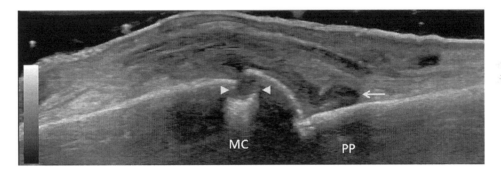

MC     PP

**Fig. 16.3** Metacarpophalangeal joint, dorsal long-axis view. Rheumatoid arthritis. Distension of joint capsule is seen (*arrow*). Bony erosion shows as discontinuity of bony contour of metacarpal head (between *arrowheads*). *MC* metacarpal head; *PP* proximal phalanx

between hyperechoic tendon sheath and hyperechoic tendon fibers. Doppler studies can show hyperemia of this synovial tissue in active inflammation.

## Bony Erosion (Fig. 16.3)

Many forms of arthritis are associated with the formation of bony erosions. Sonographically, erosions are defined as breaks in the cortical contour seen in two perpendicular planes [5]. Ultrasonography detects more erosions than conventional radiography, particularly early in the disease [6]. Bony erosions in a characteristic pattern and distribution are a hallmark feature of rheumatoid arthritis (RA). Proximal interphalangeal (PIP) joints, metacarpophalangeal (MCP) joints, wrists, elbows, and metatarsophalangeal (MTP) joints are particularly affected, often in a symmetric distribution. Ultrasonography is more sensitive than conventional radiography in detecting these erosions, particularly in early disease. In RA, these erosions are often

**Table 16.1** Bony erosion characteristics

| | Rheumatoid arthritis | Osteoarthritis | Gout |
|---|---|---|---|
| Joints most commonly effected | PIP | DIP | |
| | MCP | First CMC | |
| | MTP | Shoulder | |
| | Wrist | Hip | |
| | Elbow | Knee | |
| | | Forefoot | |
| Synovial pannus tissue | Yes | No | No |
| Other distinguishing features | No latently located erosion | Spur formation | Tophi |
| | | Centrally located erosion | Marginal bony overhang |

associated with invading synovial pannus tissue. This tissue can also be detected sonographically. Osteoarthritis (OA) is occasionally associated with bony erosions. This can then be called "erosive osteoarthritis." These erosions affect joints that are typically affected by OA, including distal interphalangeal (DIP) joints, the first carpometacarpal (CMC) joint, shoulder, hip, knee, and forefeet. In contrast to the marginal erosions of RA, the erosions of OA are often centrally located and are not associated with invading pannus tissue. Bone spur formation can be observed in the same joint. This would not be seen in RA. In gout, erosions can be associated with marginal bony overhangs, a characteristic feature of gout. Gouty erosions can be associated with tophi of monosodium urate (MSU). These tophi may be seen invading the subchondral bone [7]. Synovial pannus tissue is not a typical feature of gout.

Characteristics of bony erosion are outlined in Table 16.1.

## Enthesitis (Fig. 16.4)

Psoriatic arthritis, ankylosing spondylitis, arthritis associated with inflammatory bowel disease, reactive arthritis (Reiter's syndrome), and undifferentiated spondyloarthritis belong to the spondyloarthritides, characterized by inflammatory, erosive arthritis, new bone formation (in contrast to RA), as well as inflammation at the attachment points (entheses) of ligaments and tendons [8]. This inflammation at the entheses can be associated with new bone formation or calcification. This leads to bridging osteophytes, for example, in the case of ankylosing spondylitis. Enthesitis, one of the hallmark features of this group of diseases, can readily be assessed sonographically [9]. Blood flow at the interface of tendon and bone (a normally avascular region) can be detected with Doppler ultrasound. Edema of tendon or ligament at and near origin or insertion

appears sonographically as a loss of dense packing of parallel fibers, decreased echogenicity due to interfibrillar fluid-containing tissue, and an increased diameter. Effusion and synovial proliferation in associated synovial structures can be seen (e.g., the retrocalcaneal bursa in Achilles tendon enthesitis). Bony erosion outside of synovial joints can be seen at and near the enthesis (e.g., erosions of the posterior aspect of the calcaneus). Typically affected entheses include the common extensor tendon at the lateral epicondyle of the elbow, the origin of the patellar ligament at the distal pole of the patella, and the insertion of the Achilles tendon [10].

## Crystal Arthritis (Fig. 16.5a, b)

Gout is the most common form of inflammatory arthritis in men over 50 and postmenopausal women. It is characterized by deposition of aggregates of MSU crystals in joints and soft tissues, in patients with long-standing hyperuricemia (levels of serum urate above solubility). These tophi are surrounded by a corona of inflammatory cells and are embedded in a matrix of fibrovascular tissue [11]. Contact of tophi and their surrounding inflammatory cells with adjacent bone leads to erosion formation. Chronic, low-degree (subclinical) inflammation can lead to joint deformity over time. If this equilibrium is disturbed (sudden increase in serum urate levels through diet, sudden drop in urate level through treatment, dehydration, trauma, etc.), inflammatory cells are attracted to MSU crystals or tophi, and a gout attack ensues.

MSU crystals are strongly echogenic; they are seen as hypo- to hyperechoic aggregates of bright-appearing crystals [12]. The packing of MSU crystals in tophi allows through transmission of sound waves. Tissues deep to MSU tophi can be seen at frequencies that are used in musculoskeletal ultrasound. There is typically not a pronounced posterior acoustic shadow visible (occasionally, in very long-standing gout, tophi can become very dense or calcify, and lower frequencies are needed for assessment of structures deep to the tophi). On conventional radiographs, MSU tophi are usually not visible, but aggregates of calcium-containing crystals are. This can help distinguish gout from pseudogout due to calcium pyrophosphate dihydrate (CPPD) deposition.

In joints, MSU tophi and CPPD crystals have different patterns of distribution. In gout, MSU crystals deposit on the outer surface of hyaline cartilage. Sonographically, this creates the appearance of a "double contour" [13]. The outline of the hyperechoic bony cortex is paralleled by a hyperechoic layer of crystals, with anechoic to hypoechoic hyaline cartilage separating both. In contrast, CPPD crystals deposit in central lacunes of hyaline cartilage, so that a

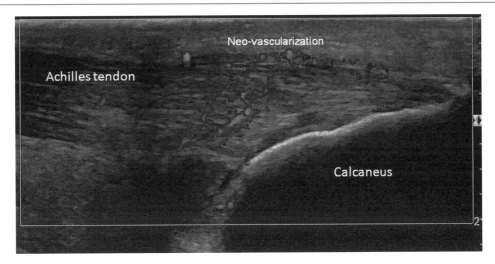

**Fig. 16.4** Achilles tendon insertion, dorsal long-axis view. Enthesitis in psoriatic arthritis patient. Hyperemia of tendon near insertion into calcaneus is seen. Areas of neovascularization appear red orange under Doppler

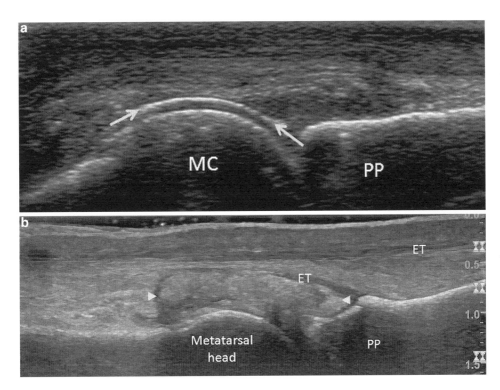

**Fig. 16.5** (**a**) Metacarpophalangeal joint, dorsal long-axis view. Double-contour sign of gout. Hyperechoic crystalline deposits over anechoic hyaline cartilage and hyperechoic bony contour are seen between *arrowheads*. *MC* metacarpal head; *PP* proximal phalanx. (**b**)

First metatarsophalangeal joint, dorsal long-axis view. Tophaceous gout. Hyperechoic tophaceous deposits distend the joint capsule (between *arrowheads*). *ET* extensor tendon; *PP* proximal phalanx

hyperechoic band of crystal is embedded in the anechoic or hypoechoic-appearing hyaline cartilage. Similarly, calcium-containing crystals may appear in the center of fibrocartilage. Typical areas accessible to sonographic assessment include the posterior aspect of the glenoid labrum in the shoulder, the triangular fibrocartilage of the wrist, and the menisci of the knee.

## Red Flags

### Synovitis

Synovitis can have different meanings: simple joint effusion without synovial thickening, thickening of the synovial lining of a joint, and synovial hyperemia. While aspiration is appropriate for simple synovial effusions, synovial thickening and particularly pronounced synovial hyperemia seen on Doppler ultrasound are signs of inflammatory arthritis. A referral to the rheumatologist for an evaluation of systemic inflammatory arthritis, including rheumatoid arthritis, would be appropriate in this setting.

## Crystal Arthritis

If typical hyperechoic, tophaceous material in or around joints and tendons is found sonographically, an evaluation for gout, and subsequent treatment, is appropriate. The evaluation may include aspiration of tophaceous material. The aspirated material can be assessed in a qualified office or in the lab with polarizing microscopy for the presence of typical crystals.

## Pearls and Pitfalls

### Gout: Double-Contour Versus Interface Reflex

In gout, MSU (uric acid) crystal can precipitate on hyaline cartilage over bony surfaces in joints. This creates the sonographic appearance of a "double contour." The hyperechoic, bright bony contour is covered by anechoic (or hypoechoic) dark hyaline cartilage. Bright, hyperechoic crystalline deposits form the second contour. This may be confounded with the bright, hyperechoic interface reflex over hyaline cartilage. This reflex is created when sound waves are reflected at the angle of perpendicular incidence off the surface of cartilage. This bright outline usually appears at the surface area of cartilage that is nearest to the transducer (if no beam steer is used). In contrast to this, the rough surface deposits of urate crystals follow the contour of the bone over a wider area. The crystal deposits create multiple small surfaces that reflect the sound waves in all directions. The reflection of the "double-contour" sign is, therefore, less dependent on the transducer position.

### Synovial Hyperemia: Artifact Versus Real Signal

Ultrasonography is particularly well suited to detect and characterize inflamed tissues [14]. Power Doppler or color Doppler signals can be seen in synovial tissues of patients who would otherwise be thought to be in clinical remission based on physical examination and serology [15]. As the gain on the Doppler mode increases, so does the area that "lights up" on the screen. Sensitivity and specificity of Doppler signals are improved if a few simple steps are followed. First, turn the Doppler setting to its maximal gain. Notice that the "Doppler box" will completely fill with

signals. Then, decrease the gain until artifacts deep to the bony surface disappear. (Ultrasonography at frequencies used in musculoskeletal ultrasound cannot penetrate bone. Any signals that appear deep to the bony cortex are therefore by default artifacts.) Finally, adjust the Doppler box to cover just a small area being scanned. This will take up less computing power and provide faster image turnover. Then, identify suspicious areas (e.g., hypoechoic synovitis) in gray scale first. Try to match any Doppler signals with this area that was identified in gray scale. Making anatomic "sense" of your signals is one of the best protections against mistaking artifacts for actual blood flow. Look for "constant" Doppler signals, and disregard signals that appear and disappear randomly. Other sources of signals that can mimic synovitis are from blood vessels and probe or patient motion. If the Doppler signal is synchronous with the patient's pulse, rotate the probe's axis to help distinguish it from small blood vessels. Anchor your probe hand against the patient or other stable object. Use two hands, and position the patient on a stable surface to avoid motion artifacts.

## Clinical Exercise

In order to appreciate abnormalities in patients, it is very helpful to familiarize yourself with normal sonographic anatomy.

The following exercises are recommended:
1. Identify anatomical structures in finger joints.
   (a) MCP joint from dorsal (Fig. 16.6). Place probe in the longitudinal or long axis over midline of MCP joint. Joint line should be in center of image on screen. Elongate the image so that the shaft of the metacarpal bone is seen on screen proximally and proximal phalanx distally. Make sure that bones do not run out of plane. Identify bony cortex of metacarpal shaft, anatomical neck, and metacarpal head. *Pearl*: The anatomic neck just proximal to the metacarpal head may be confused with a bony erosion. Erosions, however, are defined as breaks in the cortical contour. With "rocking" of the probe (i.e., proximal-distal tilt maneuver), the cortical floor of the anatomic neck can usually be seen. Identify bony cortex of proximal phalanx. Appreciate the anechoic or hypoechoic layer of hyaline cartilage over the metacarpal head. The smooth surface of cartilage can sometimes create an "interface reflex" at the angel of perpendicular incidence of the sound waves (i.e., at the portion of the cartilage that is closest to the transducer) if no beam steer is used. Overlying the dark, anechoic to hypoechoic hyaline cartilage is the fibrous tissue of the joint capsule. Over the joint space of metacarpal head and proximal phalanx, the joint capsule extends into a fibrous triangle that fills the space between the

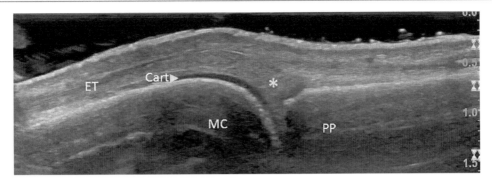

**Fig. 16.6** Metacarpophalangeal joint, dorsal long-axis view. Normal findings. *ET* extensor tendon; *cart arrowhead* hyaline cartilage; *asterisk* triangular extension of joint capsule; *MC* metacarpal head; *PP* proximal phalanx

bones. Fibrous tissue usually appears bright and hyperechoic. Due to anisotropy, this fibrous triangle may appear dark and anechoic. This could mimic a joint effusion. Try to overcome this anisotropy with rocking of the probe. Slightly adjust the angle of insonation. Creating the image of a bright triangle that fills the space between the bones will help confirm that no effusion is present. Lastly, identify the extensor tendons overlying the fibrous joint capsule.

(b) MCP joint from volar (Fig. 16.7). From volar, place the probe in long axis along the metacarpal bone and proximal phalanx, so that the joint line is in the center of the image. Identify hyperechoic outlines of metacarpal head and proximal phalanx. Find the hyaline cartilage of the metacarpal head. The volar plate is a strong fibrous stabilizer of the joint capsule that helps prevent overextension of the fingers. Superficial to the hyperechoic, bright volar plate run the flexor tendons. The flexor tendons are bound down by the A1 pulley at the level of the metacarpal head. Identify the usually dark, anechoic-appearing A1 pulley superficial to the flexor tendons. *Pearl*: Tendons and metacarpal bone are not perfectly aligned. You can often show either tendons or bones across the screen from the volar aspect.

(c) PIP joint from volar (Fig. 16.8). Align the probe's long axis along tendons and bones from the volar aspect, with the PIP joint in the center of the screen. Identify the bony contour of proximal and middle phalanx. Hyaline cartilage that lines the head of the proximal phalanx will appear anechoic or dark. The volar plate is a pronounced fibrous plate that overlies bones and cartilage and forms the joint capsule. It helps prevent overextension of PIP joints. Appreciate the tendons superficially to the volar plate. *Pearl*: Joint fluid is only seen deep to the volar plate. Fluid collections that are frequently seen superficially to the volar plate communicate with the tendon sheath, not the joint.

2. Assess vascularity of pulp of fingertip with power or color Doppler (Fig. 16.9). Assessment of increased blood flow

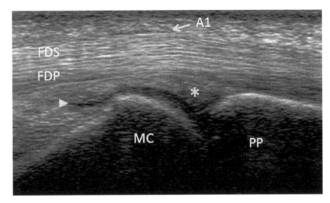

**Fig. 16.7** Metacarpophalangeal joint, volar long-axis view. Normal findings. *A1 arrow* A1 pulley; *FDS* flexor digitorum superficialis tendon; *FDP* flexor digitorum profundus tendon; *arrowhead* proximal volar joint recess; *asterisk* volar plate; *MC* metacarpal head; *PP* proximal phalanx

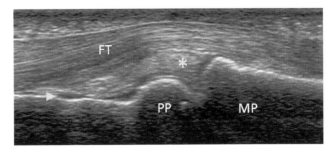

**Fig. 16.8** Proximal interphalangeal joint, volar long-axis view. Normal findings. *FT* flexor tendon; *arrowhead* proximal volar recess of joint; *asterisk* volar plate; *PP* proximal phalanx; *MP* middle phalanx

in tissues is critical for the sonographic assessment of inflammatory conditions. Distinguishing actual blood flow from artifacts may be somewhat challenging at first. It is also helpful to be familiar with the Doppler capabilities of your machine. Doppler settings may be adjusted so that the sensitivity is high enough to detect neovascularity or engorgement of smaller vessels in inflamed tissues without creating artifacts. The volar aspect of the fingertip has highly vascularized tissue, even in normal individuals.

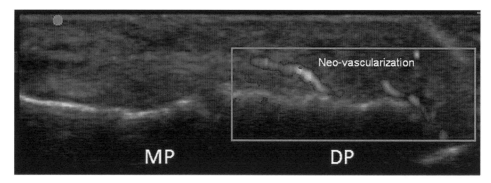

**Fig. 16.9** Volar long-axis view of fingertip. Power Doppler shows digital vessel. Areas of neovascularization appear red orange under Doppler. *MP* middle phalanx; *DP* distal phalanx

This tissue may help gauge the quality and settings of your color and power Doppler function. Place the probe over the volar aspect of your fingertip. Use very little pressure. This may be achieved by using a generous layer of gel between probe and finder, or by using light touch. Adjust the size of your Doppler box so that the pulp of your fingertip is covered, but not areas proximal or distal to it, and no significant room remains deep to the bone. With the right Doppler settings, a larger digital artery should be seen adjacent to the bony contour of the distal phalanx. Verify pulse synchronous flow to rule out artifacts.

3. Appreciate anisotropy of Achilles tendon insertion. Anisotropy occurs where sound waves meet highly reflective surfaces, particularly tendons that curve away from the transducer. Sound waves may be reflected at an angle that does not allow complete detection by the transducer, creating the false image of "missing structures." Typical examples include the biceps tendon, which can appear artificially "dark" if the tendon fibers are not aligned parallel to the transducer footprint, and the Achilles tendon, whose most distal fibers curve down to meet the bony surface of the calcaneus. To practice recognition of anisotropy as an artifact, place the transducer over the distal Achilles tendon, so the tendon fibers of the main body of the tendon run parallel to the transducer surface (footprint). The tendon fibers will appear bright, but a dark triangle may be seen at the distal attachment area. If the transducer angle is tilted down, with the distal portion moving more anterior to patient or model, the distal tendon fibers will again run more parallel to the transducer, and the anisotropy can be overcome.

## References

1. Thiele RG. Ultrasonography applications in diagnosis and management of early rheumatoid arthritis. Rheum Dis Clin North Am. 2012;38(2):259–75.

2. Backhaus M, Burmester GR, Gerber T, Grassi W, Machold KP, Swen WA, et al. Guidelines for musculoskeletal ultrasound in rheumatology. Ann Rheum Dis. 2001;60(7):641–9.

3. Mandl P, Balint PV, Brault Y, Backhaus M, D'Agostino MA, Grassi W, et al. Metrologic properties of ultrasound versus clinical evaluation of synovitis in rheumatoid arthritis: results of a multicenter, randomized study. Arthritis Rheum. 2012;64(4):1272–82.

4. Schmidt WA, Schmidt H, Schicke B, Gromnica-Ihle E. Standard reference values for musculoskeletal ultrasonography. Ann Rheum Dis. 2004;63(8):988–94.

5. Wakefield RJ, Balint PV, Szkudlarek M, Filippucci E, Backhaus M, D'Agostino MA, et al. Musculoskeletal ultrasound including definitions for ultrasonographic pathology. J Rheumatol. 2005; 32(12):2485–7.

6. Wakefield RJ, Gibbon WW, Conaghan PG, O'Connor P, McGonagle D, Pease C, et al. The value of sonography in the detection of bone erosions in patients with rheumatoid arthritis: a comparison with conventional radiography. Arthritis Rheum. 2000;43(12):2762–70.

7. Schlesinger N, Thiele RG. The pathogenesis of bone erosions in gouty arthritis. Ann Rheum Dis. 2010;69(11):1907–12.

8. D'Agostino MA, Said-Nahal R, Hacquard-Bouder C, Brasseur JL, Dougados M, Breban M. Assessment of peripheral enthesitis in the spondylarthropathies by ultrasonography combined with power Doppler: a cross-sectional study. Arthritis Rheum. 2003;48(2): 523–33.

9. McGonagle D, Lories RJ, Tan AL, Benjamin M. The concept of a "synovio-entheseal complex" and its implications for understanding joint inflammation and damage in psoriatic arthritis and beyond. Arthritis Rheum. 2007;56(8):2482–91.

10. D'Agostino MA, Aegerter P, Jousse-Joulin S, Chary-Valckenaere I, Lecoq B, Gaudin P, et al. How to evaluate and improve the reliability of power Doppler ultrasonography for assessing enthesitis in spondyloarthritis. Arthritis Rheum. 2009;61(1):61–9.

11. Dalbeth N, Pool B, Gamble GD, Smith T, Callon KE, McQueen FM, et al. Cellular characterization of the gouty tophus: a quantitative analysis. Arthritis Rheum. 2010;62(5):1549–56.

12. Thiele RG. Role of ultrasound and other advanced imaging in the diagnosis and management of gout. Curr Rheumatol Rep. 2011;13(2):146–53.

13. Thiele RG, Schlesinger N. Diagnosis of gout by ultrasound. Rheumatology (Oxford). 2007;46(7):1116–21.

14. Thiele R. Doppler ultrasonography in rheumatology: adding color to the picture. J Rheumatol. 2008;35(1):8–10.

15. Brown AK, Quinn MA, Karim Z, Conaghan PG, Peterfy CG, Hensor E, et al. Presence of significant synovitis in rheumatoid arthritis patients with disease-modifying antirheumatic drug-induced clinical remission: evidence from an imaging study may explain structural progression. Arthritis Rheum. 2006;54(12):3761–73.

# Appendix: Musculoskeletal Ultrasound Checklist

This is a general guide to assist you when scanning structures for each joint. The checklist was created using data from *Fundamentals of Musculoskeletal Ultrasound*, by Jon A. Jacobson, and from information found on the European Society of Musculoskeletal Radiology website (http:www.essr.org).

## Shoulder Checklist

- Long head biceps
- Humeral head
- Subscapularis
- Supraspinatus
- Infraspinatus
- Teres minor
- Acromioclavicular joint
- Dynamic testing of subacromial impingement
- Glenohumeral joint
- Spinoglenoid notch

## Elbow Checklist

- Anterior
  - Bicep tendon insertion
  - Anterior joint recess
  - Brachialis
  - Humeroulnar joint
  - Pronator teres
  - Nerves: median, radial
  - Brachial artery
- Posterior
  - Triceps
  - Olecranon
  - Cubital tunnel and ulnar nerve
    - Dynamic instability test
- Medial
  - Common flexor tendons
  - Ulnar nerve
    - Dynamic stress test
  - Ulnar collateral ligament
    - Dynamic stress test
    - Lateral
  - Radiocapitellar joint
  - Lateral epicondyle
  - Brachioradialis
  - Common extensor tendons
    - Extensor carpi radialis

## Wrist Checklist

- First dorsal (extensor tendon) compartment (APL, EPB)
- Second dorsal compartment (ECRL, ECRB)
- Third dorsal compartment (EPL)
- Fourth dorsal compartment (EDs)
- Fifth dorsal compartment (EDM)
- Sixth dorsal compartment (ECU)
- Radial artery
- Radial nerve
- Dorsal radioulnar joint
- Scapholunate ligament
  - Dynamic test
- Flexor carpi radialis
- Flexor carpi ulnaris
- Flexor retinaculum
- Carpal tunnel
  - FDS, FDP, FPL
  - Median nerve
- Guyon's canal (ulnar nerve and artery)
- Triangular fibrocartilage

## Finger Checklist

- MP joint
- PIP joint
- DIP joint

J.M. Daniels and W.W. Dexter (eds.), *Basics of Musculoskeletal Ultrasound*,
DOI 10.1007/978-1-4614-3215-9, © Springer Science+Business Media New York 2013

- Flexor tendon
- A1, A2 pulleys
- Extensor hood
- Thumb
  - First MCP
  - IP
  - UCL
  - A1 pulley

## Hip/Groin Checklist

- Anterior hip joint
- Femoral head
- Femoral neck
- Acetabular labrum
- Iliopsoas tendon
- Anterior joint recess
- ASIS
- AIIS
- Femoral neurovascular bundle
- Symphysis pubis
- Rectus abdominis
- Common adductor tendon
  - Adductor magnus
  - Adductor longus
  - Adductor brevis
- Rectus femoris
- Sartorius
- Greater trochanter
- Gluteus: medius, minimus, maximus
- Tensor fascia lata
- Iliotibial band
- Sciatic nerve
- Ischial tuberosity
  - Hamstring origin

## Knee Checklist

- Quad tendon
- Suprapatellar recess
- Patellar tendon
- Prepatellar bursa

- Infrapatellar bursae: infra- and suprapatellar
- Hoffman's fat pad
- Patellar retinaculae: medial and lateral
- Femoral trochlea
- Medial collateral ligament (MCL)
- Medial meniscus
- Pes anserine
- Iliotibial band
- Lateral collateral ligament (LCL)
- Lateral meniscus
- Semimembranosus tendon
- Popliteal space
- Popliteus
- Medial and lateral gastrocnemius
- Bicep femoris
- Fibular head
- Common peroneal nerve

## Ankle Checklist

- Anterior joint recess
- Extensors: hallucis longus, digitorum longus
- Tibialis anterior
- Arteries: anterior tibial, dorsalis pedis
- Anterior talofibular ligament
- Calcaneo-fibular ligament
- Peroneal tendons
- Flexors: hallucis longus, digitorum longus
- Posterior tibialis
- Tarsal tunnel
- Tibial nerve
- Sural nerve
- Achilles tendon
- Retrocalcaneal bursa

## Foot and Toes Checklist

- Plantar fascia
- MTP joint
- IP joints
- Interdigital nerve

# Index

Druck: Canon Deutschland Business Services GmbH

Ferdinand - Jühlke - Str. 7· 99095 Erfurt